TAP TALK, TIDBITS, AND TIPS FOR DILETTANTE TAPPERS

The World's Only Completely Nonessential Guide to Tap Dancing

AUTHORED BY MISTER HOLLYWOOD (A.K.A. BERNARD MICHAEL PATTEN)

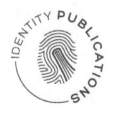

For permission requests, write to the publisher at contact@ identitypublications.com.

Orders by U.S. trade bookstores and wholesalers. Please contact Identity Publications: Tel: (805) 259-3724 or visit www.IdentityPublications.com.

ISBN-13: 978-1-945884-70-2 (paperback)
ISBN-13: 978-1-945884-71-9 (hardcover)

First Edition
Publishing by Identity Publications (www.IdentityPublications.com)

"Write whatever you like!"

– Seamus Heaney, the fourth Irishman to win
the Nobel Prize in Literature

TABLE OF CONTENTS

WELCOME

Hey there. Thanks for dropping by. And welcome.

Welcome to this little chapbook. Thank you for taking a look at it. If you picked it up, you most likely already feel you might give tap dancing a try to see if you like it and to see if it likes you. Or—perhaps—you're already into tap dancing, this major and very deep art form, and you wish to get better at it and learn more about it. Or maybe you just like tap stories the way cat people like cat stories.

You now have in hand the world's first and only tap dance book written by a student of tap and not written by a teacher, a studio owner, or an expert. Everyone suspects himself of at least one cardinal virtue, and this is mine: I am one of the few honest people that I have ever known and am therefore entirely fit to produce and write one of the few honest books about the genuine experiences of being an amateur tap dancer. Thus, we have here the world's first, best, and worst, and only completely non-essential guide to tap dancing. It uniquely tells the experiences of an amateur tapper and the true, real-life tap adventures (his and his group's), the multiple entertainments, the unique pleasures, the great fun, the frequent faux pas, and the occasional hardships. All that might or might not whet your appetite for tap dancing and might or might not give you a head's up on what to expect from tap dancing in your own life, should you decide to give it a try, or should you decide to continue tapping, as the case may be.

Either way—good!

Primarily, this book helps your brain direct your heart, nerves, muscles, sinew, and soul to serve your tap-dancing goals and to increase your tapping fun. Here you will find ideas and suggestions and discussions about dancing in general and tap dancing in particular, including the fundamental idea that dance is mainly a task of the mind and not just the body. The spirit you bring to dance is what counts the most and makes dance an edifying art form.

Here, you, the reader, will, I hope, get a satisfying mix of deep scientific fact, real research results, tap tips, tap talk, chit-chat, chatter, as well as some writing peppered with charming and amusing anecdotes. Toward the end, there is an emphasis on human memory, especially human memory applied to dancing, as well as some interesting commentary on such and related subjects. None of this will transform your life, none of this will make you excessively rich, and none of this will make you too famous.

So what?!

Who the heck wants to be too rich or too famous?!

Yes, the things here on these pages won't do a lot for you, but they should increase your fun, and that's nothing to sneeze at. Part of the fun is in meeting and getting to know new friends and people. So many people have enriched my life since I began tap dancing (so long ago) that just mentioning them would fill several pages. Thanks, you all, thanks for the memories. Most of you, my dear friends, I know are eccentric, and I have always been completely OK with that. It is all part of this wonderful and crazy tap dance experience. And yes, most of the tap teachers, viewed from a certain angle, are eccentric and obsessive and driven—by what? I don't know. Something unusual. Something a little out of joint. Something a little crazy. Probably a love of rhythm—as Gershwin said, "(For) rhythm can drive you crazy." He was joking. I think. The flipside is more likely: Lack of rhythm will drive you crazy faster. Either way, who cares? Most of us, driven by the challenge of complex tap steps and the opportunity of making music with our feet, are a little crazy. So what! I know I am a little crazy, and I can't say it bothers me. How about you?

* * *

Friends, I firmly believe we are on this planet for one purpose and one purpose only—to have fun. Some dancers are grounded, some are airborne, some are Latin based, but all have fun. Make this book only part of your dance experience and fun. Get involved with the local scene. There are many dance communities out there. In your own neck of the woods, there are likely studios and tap groups. Typically, these groups are extremely welcoming and offer a great way to meet and make new friends! Ancient Chinese wisdom: Best time plant fruit tree: Twenty years ago. Second best time plant fruit tree: Now. The best time to have started your tap career is (actually was) twenty years ago. The second-best time is now.

So, get ready to step into a fantastic way of having fun. You know, dance is more than just moving to music.

It has benefits that relate to many aspects of life usually not thought about. It is a physical activity, a creative outlet, a stress reliever, a means to mental and cognitive functioning, a way to socially engage, and an educational tool that offers insights into history and culture. Tap dance class can become much more than an activity producing noise from your shoes. Do you agree with John Lennon, who famously said, "Time you enjoy wasting was not wasted"?

How to Use This Chapbook

See what you like and see what you don't like. See what likes you and see what doesn't like you. See what works for you and what doesn't work. Take what works and then, after due consideration, discard what does not work. Each of us is a person, an individual. General advice, therefore, may or may not apply to you or your situation or life goals. Let's face it. We are all busy people. We don't have time to do everything. We must, according to our own ideas and interests, be selective and fill the unforgiving minutes with sixty seconds worth of distance run or, in this case—dancing done.

There is wisdom in the proverb "Nous sommes toujours a l'ecole." ("We are always at school."). The true finishing school is a lonely place, where within narrow walls, each one of us as individuals must learn a lifelong lesson of self-control and discipline. As a tap artist, you must seek your performance from without (known as bottom-up instruction, in which the senses dictate what comes next, and from within (known as top-down instruction), during which you turn your attention inwards and consciously direct the steps and the music from there. No book can do this for you. You must do it in your own way and at your own pace. In bottom-up, you take the clues and cues from the senses, usually how and when you hear the music or when the melody indicates the steps, or the dancer ahead of you or at your side starts a move. In top-down, you consciously control where and when you do the things you need to do, and you control directly using your willpower to make your muscles, nerves, hands, arms, and legs perform.

Examples:

Bottom-up—you hear the music and respond without thinking to do the steps at that point in the dance.

Top-down—you consciously control what you do, counting off to eight and then starting the shim-sham.

Both techniques operate in each and every performance. How and why to use each will soon be discussed.

Classic Examples of Bottom-Up Management

Forcing yourself to smile often and everywhere will actually change your brain chemistry toward a happy state. Don't believe me? Try it. Our brains copy what the body is doing. So do happy things. "Use can change the stamp of nature," said William Shakespeare, and he was right. "Put on a happy face" and "Pretend you're happy when you're blue" are quotes from the great American songbook and good advice.

The Pencil of Happiness Study

The study on this subject I like the best used a pencil to induce facial expression. If a pencil is held in the teeth, the face takes on the appearance of a smile, and the brain scans show the brain gets happy, and the person gets happy as well. If the same pencil is held in the lips and not with the teeth, the facial muscles assume positions that resemble sadness and, lo and behold, the brain scans show the changes associated with sadness, and the person tends to feel sad. Try this yourself. See if it holds true for you. Don't bite the pencil too hard. Tooth marks in a pencil are off-putting.

Experiment

Hey, how about trying an experiment? Force yourself to smile for two minutes three times a day. Let's say after brushing your teeth after meals. Smile at yourself whenever you look in a mirror. Do this for a week and then self-exam to see if you notice any change in mood. When I did this, I did get happier. Whether this was a direct effect of the practice smiling or of my imagination overworking, it is hard to say. But the result was good, and now I consider it a part (a small part) of my pursuit of happiness.

Put on a Happy Face

Researchers reporting in the June 2019 Psychological Bulletin combined data from 138 studies testing more than 11,000 people worldwide on how facial expressions influence emotions and mood. They found that smiling makes people happier, scowling makes them feel angry, and frowning makes them feel sad. Smiling had broad appeal and, although the effect was small, seemed to have an infectious nature helping other people feel happier.

Following through on this reasoning, based on no data whatsoever, it seems to me likely that looking down at your iPhone would tend to manage facial muscles toward the depression mode. Prediction: Just looking down at your phone frequently will make you feel depressed.

Botox for Depression

By using a bacterial neurotoxin to paralyze facial muscles, Botox treatments get rid of forehead wrinkle lines. The treatments make it hard to frown or scowl. That led medical researchers to the idea of eliminating negative emotional bottom-up feedback that frowns give the brain. Thus, was born a new treatment for depression. (Reference: Science: vol 372 issue 6549, page 1378, June 25, 2021)

This idea of bottom-up management of emotion goes back to the 1870s: In his seminal book *The Expression of Emotion in Man and Animals*, first published in 1872, Charles Darwin (yes, the very same famous biologist of evolution) wrote that "The free expression by outward signs of an emotion intensifies it." Darwin cataloged the six facial expressions that humans use to express the six basic human emotions and asserted that animals have similar facial expressions. Having lived with my cat, P.J.Patten, for a decade, I am sure facial expression of emotion exists in at least in one cat. —P.J.

It is interesting to note that social psychology experiments in the 1970s found evidence that even fake smiles boost a person's mood. So, what should you do if you wish to look and be happy? What should you do if you want the audience to think you are happy?

I pause for reply.

Takeaway: Smile when you dance. You will look happy, something audiences like, and you may actually get happy or happier.

The Brain Benefits from Dance

Scientific research shows that mental effort is as beneficial to the brain as physical exercise is to the body. Scientific research, believe it or not, has proven that the mental exercise of playing a musical instrument seems to decrease the chance of developing dementia, including the much-feared Alzheimer's Disease.

Whoa! What does playing a musical instrument have to do with tap dancing?

Good question.

The short answer to the question is "A LOT!"

The long answer runs as follows:

When you tap, you are the musical instrument, and the rhythmic sounds you make with your tap shoes are the music. Tapping is a unique percussive musical art that combines the life-affirming properties of dance with the abstract beauty of music. If you are a tapper, you are there right at the center of this unique musical-dance art as both a dancer and a musician. Remember that you are the musician, and you are the dancer at the same time. No other art form combines dance and music-making this way.

What did you mean by saying tapping is a percussive musical art?

Another good question.

Those of you who have suffered through a classical education know that "percuss" comes from the Latin "percutere," meaning to hit, strike, or knock. Thus, an instrument that makes music by striking something is a percussive instrument. Tap shoes make their music by hitting the floor. The piano is percussive because the musical sounds are made by the hammers hitting strings.

Drums are—you tell. Think and then tell whether drums are percussive or not.

Other percussive instruments (besides drums) are your clapping hands, the celeste, the triangle, the cymbal, and the harpsichord. The old-time typewriter was used as a percussive musical instrument. No kidding. Check out typewriter music on YouTube as an example of music from a keyboard percussive instrument of a bygone era. Jerry Lewis, when he isn't looking stupid, does a nice job with all ten fingers playing on one of those big black Royal typewriters, which I myself love to play. That black Royal gives a nice solid medium-pitched sound, and the loudness depends on how hard you hit the keys. My mom typed my father's legal documents on a Royal Standard, and I used it to type my high school papers. That Royal produced my first novel, the story of the discovery of L-DOPA (an excellent book and a great read—highly recommended), and so I became an author along with Ian Fleming and Ernest Hemingway, who also made their literature with a Royal.

Sidebar about Ernest Hemingway

Come to think on it, I have a great deal in common with Ernest Hemingway. We both love cats and daiquiris. In fact, we both guzzled them by the dozen at Cuba's El Floridita. Guzzled the drinks not the cats. The daiquiri is a drink that asks you to stop, and take time out, take a moment to enjoy life. The most momentous idea, the only serious thought I have ever had while drinking them, is "Let's order another daiquiri." And like most daiquiri drinkers, Hem and I are loose easy-going types. We are both authors, write in the same language (English), and usually use the same punctuation system, and sometimes spell the same, but beyond those things, we diverge in content, style, plot, presentation, interest, quality, moral compass, philosophy, tone, pace, sentiment, and significance. Hem won a Nobel in Literature (1954), and as for me—no Nobel yet. And, of course, Hem never ever wrote a chapbook, like this one, that is a completely nonessential guide to tap dancing. And Hem will never write such a book because he killed himself. There is a tremendous difference between the living and the dead. You may have heard that dead men don't talk. They don't write books either.

Tap Rhythms with Your Typewriter

I used the Royal to tap out the rhythm of the social dances of the era, including hustle—&1 2 3 (quick quick slow slow) and foxtrot—1 2 &3 (slow slow quick quick) and tango—1 2 &3 4 (slow slow quick quick slow). Do the same if you have an old-time typewriter.

Liberace, in my opinion, is the best typewriter musician even though he pecks away with his two index fingers on a small portable. On YouTube, you can watch The Brandenburger Symphony Orchestra score over 2,578,000 views with their version of *Typewriter*. Never have I seen a more enthusiastic audience about a symphony performance. Check it out.

The typewriter makes its best sounds when a paper is inserted, and extra sounds are filliped in by moving the lever and ringing the bell. A carbon paper gives more timbre and lowers the pitch, and augments the effects. Having a bell ring when the carriage shifts is a nice way to punctulate a typewriter musical phrase.

What the Heck Does All This Talk about Typewriters Have to Do with Tap Dancing?

The typewriter and tap shoes have lots in common: The sounds are similar, and tap dancers are known to augment their performance with claps, slaps, finger snaps, fancy cane, and hat work. Tapping on wood gives nice solid low or high pitched sounds depending on the density of the wood with overtones and timbre that vary with the type of wood and the amount of free space beneath the wood. Tapping on cement is not recommended. The sounds are scratchy, and cement is hard on legs and feet and knees, and cement will scratch your metal taps.

Different Shoes Make Different Sounds

Different metal taps by different manufacturers and the actual construction of the tap shoe also control the quality, timbre, pitch, and dynamics of tap music. Choose your shoes carefully. In fact, some tappers have several different pairs. I have three. Tap shoes are a gigantic important subject which I can't help you with. Sorry. When in doubt about tap shoes, consult your teacher or an expert tapper.

Tap and Typewriter Are Similar

Both tap and typewriter deal nicely with dynamics (amplitude or loudness), rhythm, and phrasing. Tap artists and typewriter artists are inveterate showpeople, as you will see if you watch their videos on YouTube. By the way, those old movies like *Top Hat*, in my view, do not have real tap sounds. The sounds you hear are dubbed into the soundtrack, and to my ear, they sound very suspiciously like typewriter taps. Ditto the tap sounds in some instructional CDs and videos. Someone should invent a way to amplify tap sounds similar to the way an electric guitar amplifies its sounds. Until that happens, you can bet lots of tap sounds in the movies are dubbed in.

Morton Gould

By the way, if tap is not a form of music, how come composer Morton Gould was able to write four brilliant Concerti for Tap Dancer and Orchestra? In those concerti (I recommend the Czech Orchestra CD version, and I don't recommend any of the many YouTube versions), the solo instrument is always and only the tapper, just as in a piano concerto, where the solo instrument is always and only the piano.

Great YouTube videos exist made by tapping greats. Steve Martin does a cool and excellent routine with Gregory Hines. There's one with Sammy Davis Jr. with several famous tappers. There are nice movies about tap too. One that I like is *Tap*, starring Gregory Hines and Sammy Davis Jr. Bill Robinson (yes, the man himself) stars in *Bojanges*.

Question: How Do We Know Dancing and Music-Making Is Good for the Brain?

Answer: Neuroscience, the science of the brain and nervous system, tells us so. In fact, the overwhelming neuroscientific evidence shows that directed mental activity, while decreasing the chance of Alzheimer's disease and other dementias, favorably changes the actual structure and function of the human brain. Detailed prospective blinded controlled studies of large population groups matched for age and sex, and mental function have shown that the group that is actively involved in making music or in dancing or both maintains mental function much more than the control group not involved in music-making or dancing. That's a fact, and good news for us tap dancers. References for these studies and greater detail can be found in the book *Making Mental Might: How to Look Ten Times Smarter Than You Are*.

Brain Scans Confirm Epidemiological and Longitudinal Population Studies

Magnetic resonance scans of the human brain show that just 30 minutes of actual active music practice will alter, rearrange, and grow neuronal connections. The new rewiring will last about ten days, even if there is no further practice or review. That's the physical and neurological evidence. What's the evidence from the science of psychology?

Psychological Studies Provide Massive Evidence the Brain Benefits from Use

Mountains of results from testing normal human beings have proven directed mental effort (willed effort) leads to better memory, improved clarity of thought, superior powers of concentration, better personal expression, and excellent personal presentation. This evidence is not reviewed here because it is detailed and boring and not relevant to the purpose of this book, which is to help you help yourself to better tapping. This book is a practical guide, a useful, improving book, not a scientific treatise. Too much science in a book like this might upset some readers, and some might cry, and others might even hang themselves.

Takeaway: Dancing makes mental might.

Takeaway: Dancing from memory is here to stay.

People not only prefer performance from memory, modern audiences demand it. So, if you are interested in performing tap for the pleasure of others, you must memorize the dance. There is no other way.

Tap Class

The structure of tap class depends on the teacher, the age of the students, and the desires of the people in the class. Some classes include tap barre (I got this with my two teachers Frances and Judy). Others will consist of all center floor work. Technique is, of course, important, and so is fun. My preference is for variety to maintain interest. The music is vitally important for timing, rhythm, phrasing, and excitement. My experience with classical music goes back four decades, and I have learned that there are various opinions about how music is made and understood and I have kept my mouth shut when I am told that social dancing and tap dancing have strict metronomic counts. If you think music is that robotic, listen to Julie London, whose phrases are based on rubato and humanistic variation of rhythm. Julie is (like Frank Sinatra) almost never in time with the orchestra's beat. She is following (that is actually behind time) the orchestra and vice versa, but they are rarely together. The song styling, tempo, and emphasis are all hers. This gives a much more enjoyable polyphonic type of music. If you judge her by the criterion of absolute metronome regularity, you will conclude: Julie can't sing and neither can Frank Sinatra.

Shifted Rhythms

By "shifted rhythms," it is meant the change in position in the measures of a note or group of notes. One of the most striking examples of this is found in Beethoven's Seventh Symphony, at the end of the allegro, where 1&2, 1&2, 1&2 becomes &12 in measure four. It is an old musical device used in many works and sometimes as the structural device for an entire piece. Uninterrupted repetitions of the same shift constitute what is known as superimposed rhythm, a characteristic of jazz found in the works of Irving Berlin, Vernon Duke, George Gershwin, and Jerome Kern. Frequent changes of time signature are characteristic of a certain type of modern composition, but we should not forget that folk songs of many nations occasionally show great rhythmic irregularity, and also the essence of cadenzas and recitatives is rhythmic freedom, even if not expressed by varying time signatures or tempos.

One of my teachers told me I have to dance as regularly as a human heart beats. Ha ha ha. (She was of the opinion that human heartbeats are absolutely regular and machine-like). Human hearts beat regularly only when there is a pacemaker involved. In the rest of us, heartbeat varies with respiration. Furthermore, the normal musical phrase is, in fact, usually a time period based on the respiration rhythm of a normal human. Musicians know this as a long phrasing as opposed to short phrasing that exists within a few measures. The lesson here is, if you can, put a human touch, not a robotic machine-like touch, on your tap performances.

How Long Should Tap Class Be?

The length of class is important. This usually depends on the age of the students. As for me, an hour is enough because my interest fades after an hour, and my feet hurt, and I want to go home to rest.

Pace—this is key. All steps can be faked. I know because, in the beginning, I faked a lot by just hitting the beat and moving my feet. Faked steps are not recommended. A step should not be used in performance until it is mastered and performed properly. In class, progress will be slow. Real slow. Get used to it and be patient with yourself and others.

Attitude—American teachers (unlike those in England) are relaxed and colloquial. That's the way I like them, and under that kind of teacher, I thrive. Under the teacher who is into absolute discipline, I fail to thrive. That's me. You have to pick your teacher according to your personal preferences and needs, and goals.

No audience should be subjected to poorly choreographed dances that are too difficult for the dancers. Everything should be done in due time. Only then will body, mind, feet, legs, arms, costumes, and props be all ready. Then and only then will you really "tap."

Class

For the amateur adult, the open class is the best way forward. Find a class and classmates that suit your individual needs and preferences. Something will click when the right class and the right teacher are found. And then, you, as a serious student, will start to find your own way. When we know we have a serious interest and a talent, we want to see just how far we can go with it. That is the natural thing. In my view, tap dancing is very personal—as personal and as unique as an individual's voice. Gain as much basic tap as you can from the open classes and then branch out on your own. Be an individual artist. Why not? Why not develop your style and say something different, putting your own spin on your tap dancing? Who knows, you may find yourself on a Sunday afternoon at home not copying someone else's work but developing your own artistic expression. Someone might, just might, even name after you the steps and style you invent.

Yes, name a step after you. It is possible and has happened to many others. Wipe your hand across your mouth and laugh. In my neck of the woods, we have a few Alice steps and a Noula step. Doreen Quinones has two named steps that our group does every time we do our tap version of *Cheek to Cheek*. I am not in the same league as those tappers, but I think I may have had a semi-original idea about tap that some would consider innovative.

This Is Not about a New Bernie Tap Step, as That Has Not Yet Been Invented

Ever since I was a kid, I loved to memorize and recite poems. Fifteen years ago, I discovered I could recite a poem and tap dance at the same time. The combination gave me control of tempo, phrasing, articulation, emphasis, prosody, rubato, dynamics, and so forth with interesting effects. Try this technique and see if you like it and it likes you. It isn't hard to do once you have mastered some basic steps. If you don't know a poem to recite, then tap to the Hail Mary or the Pledge of Allegiance. Don't do anything fancy—just toe-heels or flap ball changes will do to give you a feel for this form of tap. Usually, before class, when I warm up, I mentally recite some Shakespeare and tap to the rhythm and meter of his immortal noble words. For instance, consider the scene with the three witches best in Macbeth. It's question and answer time in that scene, and one witch will ask the question that the others answer.

The Tragedy of Macbeth

Act First—Scene First

1. Witch—When shall we three meet again?
    In thunder, lightning, or in rain?
2. Witch—When the hurleyburly's done,
    When the battles lost and won.
3. Witch—That will be ere the set of sun.
1. Witch—Where the place?
2. Witch—Upon the heath.
3. Witch—There to meet with Macbeth.
1. Witch—I come Graymalkin!
2. Witch—Paddock calls.
3. Witch—Anon!
    All Witches– Fair is foul and foul is fair:
    Hover through the fog and filthy air. *Exeunt.*

Poetry Tap for Your Consideration

If you wish, try to tap to this scene. Do flap ball changes, or back essences, or whatever you wish. Insert a tacet where you want. Keep the beat of the witch statements and put some drama in your recitation. Tap dancing can take it. Unsure? Confused? Take a look at Bernard Patten's YouTube channel, where he taps to the rhythm of the witches' statements.

You can dance to any poem with tap shoes on as long as you can hear it and feel it. Try this in your own home on your own floor at your own pace. Come to think on it, this opening witch scene in a very famous play (Macbeth) might make a nice tableau or an interesting skit for a show with the three witches dressed and perhaps mounting brooms to travel through the fog and filthy air. The MC should explain that a hurleyburley is a riot, that Graymalkin is the witch's cat familiar, and Paddock is the second witch's toad familiar. The familiar to a witch is a kind of special friend. The familiar of witch three is not mentioned until act 4.1, where we learn it is a harpy, a bird with talons and the head of a woman. A detailed knowledge of what is what in Shakespeare's lines makes for a much better poetry-tap experience for you and your audience. Always look up any word in the poem you are working on so you know what you are talking and tapping about.

Why Do We Tap?

Let's face it, neither I nor any tapper I know is tapping for a health benefit, and most are not even aware of the health benefit and probably could care less. At the end of the day, dance is about having fun. We are tapping for the joy of movement and the pleasure of making music with our feet. And, some of us like the lime-light and the audience adulation we get from actual performance. Me too. How about you?

Bows

And don't forget to take your bows at the end of the show. Acknowledge the applause by taking any form of bows. Correct sequence is bow first to the audience (smile too), then bow to the master of ceremonies (if there is one), and finally again to the audience before making an exit. A tapper may also acknowledge the musical conductor with a bow, and always acknowledge your partner in the duets. Good bows are as important as good performances. To bow correctly, take your time. Stand straight and then bend forward and look directly at your shoes. Ask yourself, "Are my shoes polished?" That will slow your bow and give it more dignity and power. Come up and smile directly at the audience. If the audience is hyper, wave to them. Sometimes you should even clap for the audience, especially if they were particularly moved by your performance.

Possible Benefits of Tap Dancing

Talking about benefits reminds me (interesting word—*reminds*—meaning brings back into the conscious mind) that I have received benefits from tapping that I would never have imagined possible. The temptation to tell you about these is too great so here follows my personal tap story, including how tap dancing saved my life. Decades of tap experience taught me a great deal. Some of these things may help you, and some may not. To discover which help you and which don't, continue reading.

My Story

Long ago, never mind how long, decades really, Eileen B., the ballroom dance director for our Bay Area Community Center, asked me to help her demonstrate waltz at the Pasadena Convention Center during the annual Health

Fair. The idea was to make dance look beautiful and fun in order to encourage others to join our dance club. After Eileen and I did our thing, the next act up on stage was a beautiful middle-aged brunette dressed in a red, white, and blue stars-and-stripes patriotic outfit who did a spectacular solo tap dance to the music of George M. Cohen's masterpiece *Give My Regards to Broadway*. At the point in the dance when Frances Marie Christian did trenches, the step that mimicked doughboys from World War I going over the trenches to face the German machine guns, she and tap dance had hooked me, hooked me forever. T.S. Eliot would say that I had an epiphany. An epiphany it was—an enchanted moment, face to face with something commensurate with my capacity for wonder and joy. The scene had changed before my eyes into something elemental and profound. This was the real deal: an instant wherein I became aware of a new and inexhaustible variety of activities to sweeten my life and expand my physical powers.

When Frances came down from the stage, I said, "I want to tap dance with you. I want to give my regards to Broadway." Frances turned her face to me and smiled her radiant and understanding smile as if we had been in ecstatic tap-dancing cahoots all the time.

It turned out Frances was at the health fair for the same reason Eileen and I were there. The idea was to exhibit our art and make social and tap-dancing look beautiful and fun. Eileen and I wanted people to consider taking up social dancing for the fun of it, and Frances wanted people to take up tap dancing for the fun of it. All this was and is right in line with my basic philosophy of life: We are on this planet for one purpose and one purpose only: To have fun!

In those days, Frances taught tap in the recreation room of the local Catholic Church. The group I joined had over 30 adults, two men, and 27 women. I was told, but I don't know that there was another group of about the same number of students that Frances also taught. If you are a man who wants to tap dance, make up your mind that you will be tapping mainly with women. Derek Hartley, in his six years of tap research in England (*The Essential Guide to Tap Dance, 2018*), found that 98% of tappers in-studio classes were women, a fact that matches my experiences. For me, that's good because I much prefer the society of women. I have always enjoyed a woman's company more than that of a man. Women are usually better looking and better dressed. Men are, in general, low down, deceitful, and dirty. Besides, I am a woman trapped in a man's body. In my case, I'm a lesbian, proving two wrongs can make a right.

That evening, after my first lesson, I wrote Frances an email. "Buffaloes? Time step? Shuffle? Help! I'm lost."

The reply was, "Hang in there. Come to class twice a week and sooner or later, probably later because tap is not easy, you may learn to do some simple things."

Frances was right with that *hang in there*. Persistence counts. In about six months, I could do a shuffle ball change, and after a year, my flaps, ball heels, and essence were passable. Usually, I practiced one-half hour each day, and I enjoyed the practice and enjoyed the slow but definite improvements. The major takeaway lesson was that Frances was right. Tap dance is not easy, and it is especially not easy for a middle-aged man out of shape and poorly coordinated, as I was at the time.

My mistakes were legion. Turning right when I should go left had me crashing into the dancer at my side. Often during a number I had done at least 50 times and thought I knew cold, my mind went blank. Sometimes I step on my own foot—my right hitting the left foot—when doing Irish from right to left. Once I hit my right toes with the left tap. Ouch! On rare occasions, I stepped on the dancer in front of me, usually Miss Vo. I was going forward when we were all supposed to be going back. I had problems with props, especially the cane and hats and umbrellas, often moving them at the wrong time to the wrong place with the wrong hand in the wrong way. My dressing and undressing were too slow, and that is why I needed the groupies to help keep me organized and on time. One time, I came on stage as a cowboy when I should have been dressed for my Tahitian dance.

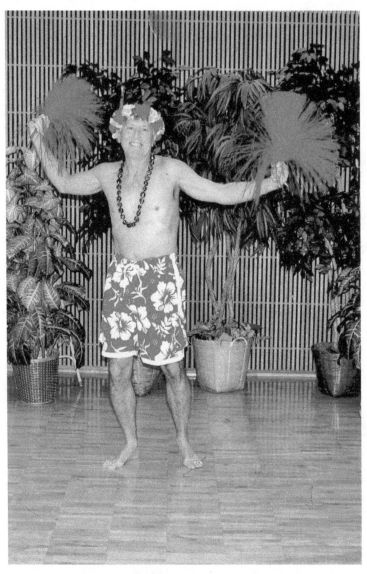

Tahitian costume courtesy of Madison Jobe Center, Pasadena, Texas.

Something went wrong with the Catholic Church, and Frances had to move our group. Frances moved us to the Beverly Hills Rec. Center and then to Strawberry Park. Those were cramped enclosed places not really suitable. We then tapped at American Legion Post 490 on Highway 3 in Webster, Texas. But the post wanted $35 for each day we were there—$70 a week. My attempts to plead our case failed. Frances taught for free, and none of us wanted to pay anything, so we had to move. Just as well because Post 490 at the time smelled unhealthy because smoking was permitted, and the place stank of cigarette smoke. I asked Nancy, the post bartender, if I could speak to Wendell (Wendell F. Denney was and still is the Post 490 adjutant and office manager) about the smell. She went back to the office, and I heard a big booming voice say, "He's a veteran and entitled to be here, but he's not entitled to talk to me."

When she came back, Nancy said, "Wendell's not here."

"Where is he?" I asked.

"Out to lunch!"

"I wanted to tell him about the cigarette smoke. Definitely unhealthy!"

Nancy shrugged her shoulders and went to the back of the bar and polished some glasses.

Frances found a home for us at the Pasadena Senior Center Madison Jobe, and we became the Silver Star Tappers of Pasadena, Texas. Now we were really set with a total wall mirror that Frances could use in a reverse way such that we students see her feet and legs the right way so we can copy her directly, and Frances sees the result without having to turn around to check our progress or lack of progress. At the barre, we worked on hard steps, cool style, elegance, speed, balance, dexterity, and adage (lyric and emotional expression).

Styling Is Important and Comes from Complete Detailed Knowledge of the Dance

If you don't think song styling is important, listen to several versions of *Blues in the Night*. Compare the style of Julie London with that of Peggy Lee. Lee's version is shorter and in jazz long-short rhythm. Lee has omitted the part B verse poem and the coda (My mama was right / my mama was right / there's blues in the night). Lee deemphasizes the long vowel sounds (cf. Julie London's singing of the words "done," "blow," and "blues"). My point is that both these singers have sung the same song, but each has a version that reflects her individual artistic vision. Each has created her own masterful rendition, which is instantly identifiable by the song styling as hers and as the work of an individual artist.

If you don't think music styling is important, take a listen to Boogie Woogie played by different pianists. It's all the same bass figure repeated rhythmically within a set twelve-measure form, but Pinetop has a light lift, Meade Lix Lewis a crashing drive, and Pete Johnson a unique "jump" style that makes all the difference.

If you think tap styling is not important, take a look at the movies of the great tappers. Notice how each has imparted their own style and personality onto the dance.

Gene Kelly's tap is as unique as his fingerprint because he used his extensive training in ballet to make his tapping incorporate parts of ballet. Fred Astaire has a more smooth ballroom look to his tap dancing. Steve Condos, on the other hand, is master of rhythmic tap. When I first saw Honi Coles tap a capella (without music), I couldn't believe he was actually moving his feet. The movements were so small, yet so effective and done without apparent effort. That day, Coles was the perfect Hoofer without any upper extremity movements at all. The immortal and famous Bojangles (Bill Robinson) style is all his own and cannot be reasonably duplicated by anyone. No wonder May 25th (Bojangles' birthday) was signed into law by President Bush as National Tap Day.

Although the truly talented old guard just cited has quit the scene and now lies on the other side of the grass, there always will be others to seek out and learn from.

My Teachers

So far in my short thirty-year tap career, I have taken tap lessons from three great teachers. Each has her own style of instruction, and each has her own style of tapping. If I were given recordings of just my tap teachers each doing the same tap dance, I would bet that I could easily tell which teacher is dancing.

Tap at Madison Jobe Senior Center Pasadena, Texas

Lou Ann Nolan was the director and very supportive with props, costumes, travel, and fun. We put on many shows for the city of Pasadena, including a Christmas show, a Veteran's Day show, Thanksgiving shows, Health Fair shows, Ms. Pasadena Senior crowning, and so forth. Believe it or not, we did nearly 40 shows a year. That was lots of practice and experience for us, and our skills grew accordingly. CNN filmed us twice, and so did local TV. During one of the TV interviews, the reporter asked me if I had any message for the people watching. I did say I get happy whenever I put on my tap shoes, but I think he probably wanted me to say something like everyone is invited to join us and have fun tap dancing, but instead, I said, "If you are watching this, you are wasting your life. Stop watching TV, and get out there and do something. Ditch the remote and grab the exercise bag. Life is what happens when you are not watching TV."

What General Activities Benefit the Brain the Most? The Short Answer.

In general, the brain benefits best from active thinking and doing, second-best from doing, third-best from thinking, and least from watching. Thus, our spectator culture is actually wasting brain power.

Just watching and not doing or not thinking is just about the worst thing you can do for your brain's health and happiness. That's why so many neurologists (myself included) hate TV—It's just junk food for the mind— empty content without intellectual value in the same way that junk food is empty calories without nutritional value. In fact, your brain is less active while passively watching TV than it is while sleeping. So given the choice, don't watch TV—Take a nap.

29

But what about educational programs on PBS and TV of that ilk?

Next time you watch such programs, pay attention to two things: The information density and the content. You may find that the information density is slight and that the content does little more than entertain you by flattering your ego by showing you stuff you already know. One Disney producer explained this to me directly: "The public will not tolerate anyone showing them stuff they are not already familiar with. The public wants affirmation that they already know all that they need to know. Try to teach them something new, and your chance of staying in business is close to zero."

Opportunity Costs: Lost Opportunities Are Opportunities Lost

The other problem with TV is that the time spent watching it could have been better spent thinking or reading or learning or playing a musical instrument or playing chess or bingo, social dancing, tapping or doing anyone of a number of activities. Any one or any combination of those activities has been shown by neuroscientists in prospective, controlled, blinded, long-term studies to augment brain power and reduce the chance of dementia. Watching TV, on the other hand, has been shown (I am not making this up) to increase your chance of developing heart disease, diabetes, cancer (cancer of the colon in particular), obesity, and dementia. TV has been shown to seriously degrade attention span and memory capacity. The average attention span of the average American, believe it or not, is less than two minutes. Significant evidence indicates that watching TV causes autism in some cases and that stopping TV stops the autism in those cases.

TV May Cause Violence

On TV, Bishop Sheen said TV causes violence. What evidence he offered, I don't recall, but I don't think Bishop Sheen would lie. Bishop Fulton J. Sheen was extremely popular in my Irish Catholic family. His show *Life is Worth Living* in the early days of TV served to introduce Americans to Catholic thought in a time when many Catholics were considered to be nefarious agents of the Pope. Rumors were circulating that a special trans-Atlantic tunnel was being constructed from the Vatican to the White House so the Pope could visit JFK! No kidding! Political discourse in America can be that stupid. It still is.

If you have time, take a look at Fulton's show on how to improve your mind. He starts out with all smiles and lots of jokes. "There is that old question if you were on a deserted island and could have one book, what would it be? Fulton pauses and smiles. He is waiting for our answer. Of course, we all think the answer is the bible. Nope. His answer is Thomas' on *How to Build a Boat*. "And then there was the man who read about the possible association of cigarette smoking and lung cancer. So, he decided to give up (smile and long pause)—reading."

Fulton won two Emmy Awards as *Most Outstanding Television Personality*. My father and mother thought he was a saint. If that was what saints were like, we all wanted to go to heaven to enjoy the company of the likes of him. Fulton was funny too, even about religious things:

31

"Hearing nun's confessions is like being stoned to death with popcorn." "There are 200 million poor in the world who would gladly take the vow of poverty if they could eat, dress, and have a home like (sic) I do."

But what was his secret? Why was he so popular? Look at the old shows, and you will see right away that he was usually smiling with open, inviting body posture and a twinkle in his eyes. That infectious boy scout smile will endear anyone. He had enthusiasm and energy, and, except when writing on the blackboard, he had direct eye contact with the audience. From his example, we dancers learn to do the same: Smile, have enthusiasm, open body postures and energy, and look directly at our audience. There is no doubt in my mind that most people in the audience want to love you. Give them the chance, and give them the look to help them.

How Much TV Do Kids Watch?

Nielsen Company says in a study released October 26, 2009, that children ages 2 to 5 watch more than 32 hours of television each week (Wall Street Journal, October 27, 2009, page A4). Kids 6 to 11 spend a little less time in front of the TV screen—more than 28 hours. But that is partly because they have to go to school. TV isn't called the electronic babysitter for nothing. Think of all those young brains that are not getting the exercise that they need for proper development. Think about all those young muscles that are not getting the exercise they need for proper development. Think of all that wasted life.

Kids Who Watch Too Much TV May Have Interesting Adverse Consequences

"Adverse consequences" is British for side effects. In America, drugs have side effects. In the U.K., there are consequences. The Guardian reported about a phenomenon among American preschoolers called the Peppa Effect. The children who watch a lot of Peppa Pig during the pandemic lockdown have developed British accents and started using British terms like "mummy" (mommy), "give it a go" (try it), and "satnav" (GPS). Wall Street Journal reporter Preetika Rana wrote that her niece "had an American accent before the pandemic. Now she has a POSH (port out starboard home) English accent." One respondent agreed: "And for Christmas, I had to put out a freaking mince pie for Father Christmas, or, as we call him here in the States, Santa Claus.

I don't know, but I think some of those kids were speaking British just to irritate their parents. When my brother and I wanted to get my mother's goat, we turned on the British, which we learned aboard the Cunard Ocean Liners as we crossed the North Atlantic. Mom would shout us down, "Stop talking like that. People might think you're fags!"

The Official Position of the American Academy of Neurology Is against TV

And so the austere, usually laconic, and rarely committed American Academy of Neurology has come out against TV as detrimental to the brain. If the neurologists don't know what's good for the brain and what isn't good for the brain, who does?

What Activities Are Best for Your Brain? The Long Answer.

The long answer to the question about which exercises are best to help the brain memorize and perform is this project and the advice, exercises, expositions, demonstrations, and techniques contained herein. Such exercises, expositions, demonstrations, and techniques evolved from the author's medical research and experience with patients that has spanned over four decades. They also derive from the author's rather limited experience as a tapper. These ideas should help you help your brain. They should, in fact, help a lot.

Silver Stars

Pictures of the Silver Stars appeared in the Citizen, Galveston News, and other local papers and sometimes even in the Houston Chronicle. We did shows at churches and nursing homes and day care centers and retirement homes and community centers and at the YMCA, Festivals like Christmas in July, and anyplace that would have us. We were in our hay day.

Audience size varied from 30–40 to over 800. No kidding. Reception was always enthusiastic despite my many flubs. As I was the only male dancer after Rufus died, and the retirement home crowd was mainly women, I was the natural center of attention and adulation. Some of my fellow tappers complained, "How come, Bernie, you are the one who usually gets all the attention."

"It's only natural, like sniffing the breeze when a steak is cooking—an animal thing. Sex appeal! Women

34

like men. The same will happen to you all if and when you transition."

About Men in Tap

It is a gigantic mystery to me why there are not more men in tap class. Men don't like the idea of learning something new because they want everyone to think they know it all already. They also are afraid to struggle, or maybe they think tap is not macho enough. Who knows? Their attitude is, in my view, very restricting, and I feel sorry for them. Tap dancing is historically a man's dance designed to make lots of noise as a drumming in the soul, a kind of loud expression of the psyche. For me, it is a way of letting people know I am still around. The men who do tap are often individualists who often like to do things out of the ordinary. Those men are not afraid of looking silly. Men, swallow your ego and get in touch with dance and music. You will probably have the same uplifting experiences I get every day I tap dance. Why miss out on feelings of happiness, personal accomplishment, and even joy? Why cheat yourself? Learn to tap, and you will be able to put on your pants while still standing. With tap experience, you will acquire that resourcefulness of movement and formless grace that is so peculiarly American. And while drunk, you will still be able to walk a straight line. And who knows, next time you fall off a roof, tap may save your life!

Tap Dancing Taught Me a Big Lesson: Avoid the Fate of Nursing Homes If You Can

The current state and conditions at some of those nursing homes were not good. People were crowded into little rooms for their meals and for sleep. No wonder the pandemic hit those places hard. Looking out at the audience, I realized there was lots of undiagnosed neurological disease out there and many other unmet needs. Before I had taken tap and seen the nursing homes first hand, they were invisible to me. Now I know nursing homes are poorly run, over and under-regulated, and understaffed by people who are undertrained and underpaid.

Say NO to a Nursing Home

Sad to say that in America, 1 in 3 people over 65 end up in a nursing home because they need long-term care. Five culprits are behind the nursing home glut—falls, heart disease, Alzheimer's, stroke, and incontinence. Try to cheat the odds and live happy and healthy to a "ripe old age" at home. The major preventable thing is to prevent falls. No kidding! You can do this!

During my 42 years in medical practice, I witnessed terrible consequences of falls even among fellow physicians who thought they could easily descend their office stairs without holding on to the rail. Every 20 minutes, a senior in America dies due to a fall. The red-hot danger zone is any room with slippery surfaces, with the bathroom leading the list. The biggest risk in the bathroom is getting in and out of the tub or shower. Sorry, but as a physician, I can't resist giving the following advice: Get rid of throw rugs, install handrails on all stairs— inside and out, secure all lamp cords, so you don't trip over them, light up your home with switches on the top and bottom of the stairs, and always use night lights to light your way safely to your bathroom. Make sure you are holding onto something solid as you enter or exit the shower or bath. My tap dancing has given me the agility of a squirrel so that when I do trip, I, thus far, have always made nice easy recoveries. Tap dance will probably do the same for you if you keep at it. All the tap dance friends I know have a physical agility that far exceeds that of normal.

Survival Is the Name of the Game. Live Independently as Long as Possible.

At the nursing homes, I realized I was looking at the future, perhaps even looking at my future because someday, I would probably be in a nursing home. But, perhaps, if I were lucky, I might be out there in a wheelchair or a walker looking at a real live tap show and cheering the dancers on while keeping time with their beat by tapping with my hands and feet. Come to think of it, that fate isn't as bad as having the dew and the green grass above me. But it does have an appointment in Samarra kind of flavor.

Appointment in Samarra? What's that?

A nice short story about fate by W. Somerset Maugham (1933). The speaker is Death herself. Here is the version I like:

There was a merchant in Bagdad who sent his servant to market to buy provisions, and in a little while, the servant came back, white and trembling, and said, "Master, just now when I was in the marketplace, I was jostled by a woman in the crowd, and when I turned I saw it was Death that jostled me. She looked at me and made a threatening gesture. Now, lend me your horse, and I will ride away from this city and avoid my fate. I will go to Samarra, and there, Death will not find me." The merchant lent him his horse, and the servant mounted it, and he dug his spurs in its flanks, and as fast as the horse could gallop, he went. Then the merchant went down to the marketplace, and he saw me standing in the crowd, and he came to me and said, "Why did you make a threatening gesture to my servant when you saw him this morning?" "That was not a threatening gesture," I said. "It was only a start of surprise. I was astonished to see him in Bagdad, for I had an appointment with him tonight in Samarra."

The lesson is clear. We can't avoid our fate. All of us, sooner or later, will be pushing up daisies. Bill Gates and Warren Buffet, who have bank accounts resembling the national debt, can't buy a second of time. And neither can you, dear reader. Use your time wisely. Do the things you want and pass up what you don't want.

God's Waiting Room by B. Patten
I see them when we tap at their nursing home
They hobble in on one stick or two
Some push walkers and others wheel wheelchairs
Then, they sit staring blankly into space
They're here, but where are their minds?

What are they thinking? What thinking?
For God's sake, don't they realize
It's not cool to piss your pants
Or hang your jaw and drool?
Don't they see what's happening?
What's happening to them?
Jesus!
They should be screaming!

Conclusion: Another really big need of nursing home residents was for something to do or to see. The bulk of the inhabitants is starved for excitement and for attention and affection and human touch and contact. They are wasting their precious time and lives. How sad! We have to do better by these neglected people. But how?

Men Dancers Have Problems at Some Nursing Homes

Yes. No questions about it. Our shows were a very big deal for the inmates (I mean residents) of the nursing homes. There were problems, though. Shows at the retirement home for nuns had to be discontinued because the nuns were too aggressive to Rufus and myself, the two male dancers. This was no big deal for me, but it did bother Rufus, and he vetoed any more shows for retired nuns. Nuns had labored too long in the vineyard of the Lord and, although each was married to Jesus and had a ring to show for it, they probably did not get enough or even any *you-know-what*.

After the show, our custom was to go through the audience and shake hands and thank them for coming.

After one performance in Deer Park, one overly made-up woman in a wheelchair motioned me over. This tawdry beauty said, "Why does your shirt say, dunce?"

"Madame, it says dance, not dunce."

"Come closer so I can read the shirt."

I came closer and pushed my chest forward, so the shirt was in front of her wide blue eyes.

And then she goosed me while screaming, "I know what this is. I know what it's for."

After that episode, Margaret decided she would protect me from the likes of that woman. From then on, at the end of the show, when we went through the audience to greet and thank them, Margaret stood between me and the women. That simple trick solved the problem.

And yes, after about eight years of tapping, Frances and I did a duet to *Give My Regards to Broadway*. We were quite a hit, and I loved the admiration of the crowds. Joy Nall and I did a wonderful tap duet to the fast and furious music of *Big Band Boogie-Woogie*. Joy was 83 at the time, and at the end of the dance, she would run, make a sudden leap and fling herself backward, landing in my outstretched arms. We did this hundreds of times, and I never failed to catch her, and I never, ever grabbed her tits. Joy said, "That is nothing to brag about, Bernie. My tits are so small they are hardly there."

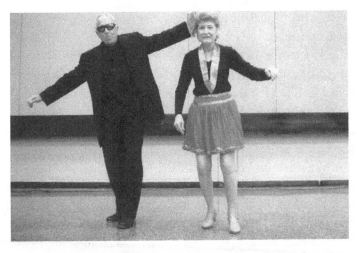

Joy and Bernie do their signature Boogie-Woogie at the Pasadena Convention Center, 2015. Notice how we as partners are still expressing our individual personalities both in costume and style.

How Tap Saved my Life

One dark, dull, drear December, I was putting Christmas lights on the roof of our home in Seabrook. My feet slipped, and I fell backward. For a brief moment, I was in the air supine facing the sky and headed to hit the ground with my back and head. Somehow, I twisted and became vertical and faced the street away from the house. The fall was about 20 feet, so I expected to break something, and I put out my right leg as that leg is my strongest body part. Bang! Thud! I hit the grass with that leg and bounced back into the air, landing another eight feet away from the house. Nothing was broken, nothing was torn, nothing was hurt. Never again will I hang Christmas lights or go on the roof. In my opinion, tap had saved my life by making me as agile as a squirrel.

Frances was not convinced. Even though I cited evidence that tap dancing had built up my foot pads so thick that I felt like I walked on air. And my leg muscles had become gigantic and powerful. The connective tissues had thickened about my ankles, and the ilio-tibial band (on the lateral side of the leg) now felt like a band of steel and not like a normal human tissue. No kidding.

My coordination had also vastly improved. Before tap, I had to sit to put on my pants. Now I put them on standing. Even when very drunk, I could stand indefinitely on either foot, and I could easily walk a straight line and look sober. All these things tap had done for me as a sort of side effect. You may get the same benefits. But don't test yourself when drunk the way I did. You might get hurt, and getting drunk is, in general, not a good idea, especially if you do not have an Irish liver as I do.

Oh, yeah, I forgot to mention the speed and grace of my walking improved. It was as if I was not walking but rather floating along. People said I walked like John Travolta, and yes, it was that walk that most real dancers acquire.

About walking: Nurses complained that I was walking too fast on rounds and, Vanessa, a fat one, had trouble keeping up. The nurses also thought I looked younger, and one of them (Velma Adams) examined the back of my neck for the scars of a facelift she was sure I had got. She found no scars. Conclusion: The nurses thought I looked ten years younger. Neither I nor they could explain why. It may have been a side effect of tap dance and the exercise and stress-reducing qualities that go with tap dancing. See if you get a similar benefit.

"Frances, in my opinion, tap prevented me from a serious injury from the fall. What's your take?"

Frances: "Irish luck! God gives the Irish this tremendous luck to make up for their tremendous stupidity and to level the playing field against the Jews. You were stupid to be on the roof and just lucky to hit the ground right. Tap may have helped, but not that much. You are definitely in good shape—for a gomer."

Frances distributed typed notes on each dance. These were written in a kind of code that we eventually understood. Here's an example:

HONKY TONK

(Moving forward)

R step, clap, L step, clap, R step, clap, L step, clap;

R flap heel, L flap heel, R step, L shuffle, L shuffle, L shuffle;

L step, clap, R step, clap, L step, clap, R step, clap;

L flap heel, R flap heel, L step. R shuffle, R shuffle, R shuffle.

At no time did Frances ever use or look at the notes while she taught us. She had memorized all the steps and all the parts of the dance she was teaching. She never called out. So, none of us were ever worried about being personally drawn on the carpet. If she saw someone doing something that needed correction, she stopped the lesson and demonstrated what was correct as if the group needed instruction and not an individual. That took the heat off because most of the women feared being embarrassed in front of the group.

Before each lesson, Frances reviewed a basic tap step and had us practice it at the barre. When I had trouble, she came right next to me and worked with me until I got it. She didn't say anything. She just repeated the step. It was show not tell. Eventually, we all had a repertoire of basic steps that were fundamental parts of most of the dances. These basic steps are the chunking tools that will help you memorize your performance dances. About that more later.

My happy tap life continued for a while until Frances got ovarian cancer in 2005. She had several courses of chemo and went into partial remissions. The chemo took its toll, and so did the cancer. Frances became less and less able to tap. Imagine the tragedy of this! A tragedy of the first magnitude and dimension. For a while, she taught from a chair, but eventually, that failed. Her daughter, Linda, returned the Rusty Frank oak tap mat I had given Frances, and that is how I knew we were close to the end. Frances was no longer practicing at home. She couldn't.

One cold December night (December 11, 2009, to be exact), Frances died, age 67. Frances was known to us as "Twinkle Toes" because of her love of tap, jazz, ballet, square dance, clogging, whip, ballroom, and especially Argentine tango with her husband, John. She had been elected Ms. Pasadena Senior in part because of her dancing skills and, according to Lou Ann Nolan—coordinator of the judges that year, "beautiful and great legs." Frances had won many local and national awards for the same reason. But goodbye to all that. It all ended with her death. Sic transit gloria mundi, (Thus passes the glory of the world.)

The boast of heraldry, the pomp of power,
And all that beauty, all that wealth e'er gave
Await alike th' inevitable hour
The paths of glory lead but to the grave.
Thomas Gray

On December 15, 2005, there was a mass at Saint Frances Cabrini Catholic Church with service by Father Frank Fabj. I always feel better when someone is delivering a eulogy, and I am listening to it. That is one of the ways I know I am not dead. Miss Vo, a boat person from Vietnam and a lead tapper who usually danced in front of me, and whom I usually copied, and sometimes stepped on, sat with me in the last row of the church listening to Father Frank's now frank (PUN intended) discussion of Jesus's horrible death on the cross.

Miss Vo spoke fluent Vietnamese but her English—"not so good." She whispered: "What did the priest just say? Something about blood."

Me: "He said unless you eat Jesus Christ's flesh and drink his blood, you cannot enter the kingdom of heaven."

Miss Vo: "Drink blood—That's disgusting!"

Two weeks later, Mis Vo (I never learned her first name if she had one. She wanted to be addressed simply as Miss Vo) quit tap because she wanted to use the time to make more money at the nail salon where she worked. Subsequently, most of the tappers left. They missed Frances, and without Frances, things weren't the same.

After mass, we said goodbye to Frances. The coffin was open, and she had on her *Give My Regards* outfit and her tap shoes. In with her were her white parasol show umbrella and one of those nice white canes she had made for herself and for us students. Severio Gaudiano, her brother, said burial with the tap stuff was Frances' last wish. "I guess she wanted to have the equipment nearby if needed."

The stuff will be there with her until judgment day, when Gabriel blows his horn. But, Jesus, did Frances look terrible—like a malnourished Asian, wretched, wasted, withered, wizen, wrinkled, and shriveled. Death is ugly. Never before had I realized death could make you look so bad. Frances was like *She* in the 1887 H. Rider Haggard novel *She: A History of Adventure*. When **She** (aka Ayesha, a 2000-year-old woman who looked marvelous for her age) pushed her luck and got in the Pillar of Fire a second time, *She* showed her true age, and her body shrunk and withered away. In short, *She* turned into a corpse and then a skeleton. The sight is so shocking that Job, one of the main characters in the book, dies in fright. Looking at what was left of our once vibrant Frances, I could understand what happened to Job. He died of fright when he saw what death could do. Ursula Andress is a great **She** in the 1965 movie, which pretty much follows the book except in the movie Job the man servant doesn't die.

Frances may be tapping in heaven or some better place. I miss her and her smile, her voice, and her intense interest in each and every student. And I am not alone. Many others miss her too.

Talking of Death Reminds Me of a Cross-Examination Done at a Trial

"Doctor, when did you start the autopsy?"

"Exactly 8:30 PM."

"And was Mister Denton dead at the time?"

"If he wasn't dead, then he certainly was when we finished."

"Doctor, how many autopsies have you performed on dead people."

"All of them were dead. The living put up too much of a fight."

"Doctor, did you check Mister Denton's pulse?"

"No."

"Did you check his blood pressure?"

"No."

"Did you check his respirations?"

"No."

"Did you check reflexes?"

"No."

"Doctor, in view of the fact you did not check those things, isn't it possible he was still alive?"

"No."

"No?"

"Yes, no. His brain had been removed and was on the table."

"But Doctor, isn't it possible Mister Denton was still alive even though his brain had been removed?"

"Yes, I suppose it is possible, and he could be still out there somewhere practicing law."

"Doctor, one last question: Isn't it true that if Mister Denton died in his sleep, he wouldn't know he was dead until the morning?"

"You know, I am having trouble believing you passed the Bar exam."

Silver Stars after Frances Died

After Frances died, most tappers left the group for many different stated reasons (knee problems, boredom, disappointment that Frances wasn't there to cheer us on, and so forth). But I think the real reason was that the routine and the dances weren't what these people were used to. Things had changed, and some people didn't like the change and couldn't adjust to the new situation. I have seen this before. A group derives energy and purpose from a given person, and then when that person leaves the scene, the group falls apart. It is as if the person was a needed catalyst to keep the chemistry going. Conclusion: The Silver Star Tappers had a certain energy and without Frances lacked a certain element supplied by her, and therefore the group changed and dissolved.

With Frances gone, Judith Grace took over teaching us. She changed almost everything. We started doing duets and tapped to songs such as *Make Someone Happy* and *Look on the Bright Side of Things* and *Colors of the Wind*. All these had inspiring happy lyrics, and in my opinion, we, the Silver Stars, actually approached a semi-professional level of theater. We certainly learned adage, dance with lyrical and emotional expression. Part of the effect was due to arm and cape control and to the multiple changes of clothes and the many new highly creative dances, all originally choreographed from scratch by Judy. Stage directions were log numbers more complicated, and we mastered some very complex scenes, which Judy said she had always dreamed of organizing, teaching, and performing.

I continued to have slips. And I continue to have slips. But my current slips are not the same, nor are they as serious, and, more importantly, my ability to hide the slips and my ability to recover has vastly improved. I am convinced that all of our shows had a fair share of misses, near-misses, and faking. This is not to suggest that we should strive toward imperfection, but we need to work as inhabitants of an imperfect world. For some reason, probably based on my vast experience as a public speaker, I never got stage fright, and that put me in a position to help others overcome their fright, some of which was disabling. I would like to suggest that in order to conquer stage fear-related problems, we must accept that perfection is, while desired, nearly impossible.

About Perfection—Not Needed. Instead, Strive for Human Expression

Yo-Yo Ma (the American cellist) told us in his master class about an interesting and important experience he had during a concert. He was playing along and thinking how perfect his performance was. Suddenly he realized that he was "bored out of my mind." Then and there, he had an insight that would change the rest of his life. Yo-Yo Ma discovered that perfection should not be the goal. The goal is to share something with others. He calls these things shared "magical moments" wherein something, an idea, a feeling, an emotion, or "something I can't say in words" is transferred to another human. At that moment in the concert, Yo-Yo Ma resolved not to seek perfection but instead to seek "human expression." He said his music and music, in general, was just a subset of all the things that can be done to establish a human connection through human expression. This little chapbook is no place to discuss in detail this philosophy of life, but many human activities such as smiling, laughing, sharing love or a good meal, or telling a joke or an amusing story (and even writing a tap book) can be viewed as beneficial human expression. Think about this: Suppose God does not exist. Then we humans have no one to rely on or to get help from but ourselves and our fellow humans. Tap dancing, I firmly believe, is a form of sharing many things with others—fun, joy, movement, friendship with ourselves, and when we perform, we are sharing our joy and happiness with the members of the audience who are reacting back and sharing their happiness with their cat-calls, claps, stomps, and hoots. Yo-Yo Ma would consider tap dancing a small but important subset of all the things we can do to create human expression and promote human connections. If everyone followed this philosophy, the world would be a much better place.

How to Exit Your Performance

Always have an exit strategy and a method in mind to handle mistakes. Besides, it is clear to me, audiences are very forgiving, and they don't care, and most wouldn't even recognize a flub or mistake. So, just ignore them and certainly never acknowledge a mistake. As long as you keep smiling and are close to hitting the beat and moving and acting like everything is OK, the audience will think everything is OK. They are always grateful to be entertained by real tappers dancing in real 3D. The Silver Stars did have an encore, which we used only when the audience was exceptional. After the encore, exit gracefully and quickly, bowing and waving and smiling your way out.

Correction

Ugh! I was wrong. Some people in the audience do notice things that most people miss. After one performance at Village on the Park, Friendswood, Texas, whose motto is "Where the Fun Never Sets," a very old woman (100+) came up and said, "You are usually a fraction of a second behind the other dancers, so you must be copying them."

"Exactly right! And very astute! Have you had dance experience?"

"In my salad days, I was a Rockette."

Stage Fright

Children do not have this problem. They are used to making mistakes and take them in stride. Ever see a two-year-old learning to walk? He falls, trips, recovers, laughs, and keeps on trying. With adults, it can be a different story. Some adults may look confident on the outside, but inside they are a mess of panic when it comes to performing in public, whether in studio for their teacher and fellow students or for family and friends at home.

Adults need to be assured and often reassured; they need to know in their deep hearts core that a mistake is not a total failure. In my view, mistakes don't matter at all. They are gone instantly. What does matter is that we are, as adults, sharing something beautiful with fellow students and with the audience. So, adults: Put your tap performance in perspective. Relax. It is not brain surgery! Do your best and be easy on yourself. But do focus your brain on the complex skills with which your body needs to deal. Master as many tap steps and techniques as you can.

Some Ideas to Prepare Adults for Performance

Perform in your own home to sympathetic friends and family. That gets you in the groove of tapping before a group. Do this before cocktails! The cocktails, even one, tend to throw me off balance, and off-balance tends to injure my feet and knees in the process. Drinking and driving is a no-no. Drinking and tapping is a no-no.

For your informal performance at home, select a dance you know very well and feel completely at ease in doing. This builds self-confidence for your cruise ship performances and your shows with your group. If I don't know the entire dance, I will just do the parts I know well. Most people will not know or care that the dance is less than it is. It is important that you know your true level of performance. Test yourself. If you can say out loud all the steps and in the correct order, then you are sure you know the dance. Some dancers will even write out each and every step as a kind of self-test. You will be surprised at how many mistakes you make and how many omissions, and how many incorrect sequences you make. Human memory is frail, and forgetting is the default mode. Don't lie to yourself about your true level of preparation. Make sure you know the dance cold. That is the best preparation and the best security against going blank during the real show. Mental review is helpful, and you can do it most places without your tap shoes on. While waiting to check out at the grocery store, I am thinking about the steps and sometimes actually tapping them with my street shoes. Others in line may think this queer, but so what? If there are places you are lost, steps you can't do, or things you question, ask your teacher or your friends for help. Don't be shy. Experience counts. After you have done 30 or 40 shows, you will feel quite at home on the stage doing your thing.

Margaret used to be a bundle of nerves before we did our duet, *Tea for Two*, but after 60+ performances, the stage fright had vanished, and she, real relaxed, was able to focus on the artistic expression of the dance. Joy Nall, an experienced dancer, never ever had any nervousness about the dance or my catching her final leap, proving individuals have individual reactions to situations. That duet to big band, as mentioned, was great fun, but I especially like dressing up as Carmen Miranda (with fake tits and an augmented butt) and doing a solo at the end of Latin dance Judy had invented.

At a local Baptist church, after the performance with me as Carmen, two men came to the dressing room. Jeanine Jones, my social dance partner and one of my groupies, answered their knock and yelled up to me. "Two men are here and want to know if you are available for dating."

I shouted, "No!"

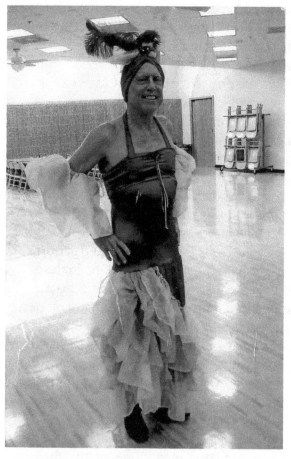

Doctor Patten's Carmen costume was designed and made by Jeanine Jones and her friend Pat, both loyal and trusted groupies.

Yes, I had groupies. Doesn't everyone?

Besides innovation in dances, music, costumes, duet, and individual dances, Judy Grace got the idea we could make money by charging for the shows. At first, a bowl was put out with a sign that asked for dollars for gas. At the more well-to-do retirement homes like Eagle's Trace, that bowl usually ended up with hundreds of dollars. Judy paid the dancers $35 each, and thus we became professional. During the many changes of costume, Judy's husband Glenn told jokes to keep the audience awake. At a contest of amateur performing groups at George R. Brown Convention Center in downtown Houston, we did our show with multiple numbers and took first place. There was a money prize, I think, and, I think, Judy kept it. For the rest of us, our reward for winning was we got to do a special show at the Westin Hotel in the Galleria. Westin built a special wood resonant tap floor for us, and we tapped for the convention of directors of Senior Centers of the State of Texas. Margaret and I did our signature duet to *Tea for Two*, but something unusual happened just before we started. Margaret looked out over that vast and eager audience and asked me, "Where are we? What's happening?"

"Margaret, we are at the Westin Hotel and are about to do our signature duet *Tea for Two*."

"*Tea for Two*? What's that?"

Ugh! Just as I thought we would have to leave the stage, the music started, and Margaret and I did a perfect exhibition of duet tapping, which was followed as usual by thunderous applause and a standing ovation. Sadly, that was the beginning of Margaret's decline into dementia.

Eventually, she was no longer there mentally, but she was still there physically. How sad! She looked like Margaret, alright, but she wasn't really Margaret. Eventually, she didn't recognize me or her other fellow tappers. It was interesting that in our last performance, the music triggered her memory, and she did the dance without much conscious thought. Several examples of this phenomenon are available on YouTube where an obviously confused and demented woman appears dazed on stage, is shown a piano and doesn't know what it is or what it is for, and then touches the keys and plays a Chopin prelude in C minor perfectly from memory. At the time Margaret dropped out of the Silver Star Tappers of Pasadena, Texas, we were six in number. Joy Nall, Ester, Judy Moody, Judy Grace, Elain Bischof, and myself. Judy Grace told us she wanted to be the teacher, and we agreed.

Ugh! You may have noted Rufus was missing. I forgot to tell what happened to him. One day at Madison Jobe tap practice, Rufus got short of breath after the warm-up and told me he couldn't continue tapping because he didn't have the energy. He felt the worst he had ever felt in his life. He sat out the rest of the lesson. If a patient had told me something like that in clinic, they would have been admitted to the hospital for evaluation. And if they refused hospitalization, I would have advised them to go home and plan their funeral. Boy, did I miss the diagnosis in Rufus!

A few days later, Rufus went to one of those Doc in a Box places. They missed the diagnosis too. They said his nausea and vomiting and stomach aches were due to food poisoning from the Tex-Mex restaurant Rufus had eaten at a few days before. The next day, his ex-wife tried to phone him and got no answer. She found him dead with his head in the toilet. He was probably trying to vomit. Cause of death: Acute myocardial infarction. Those posterior inferior infarctions do cause stomach pain, nausea, and vomiting. In retrospect, this was a classic case. There is a legend in the medical profession that the short men get the heart attacks and the tall men do not. Rufus was very short—another reason I should have been on the alert. Sorry, Rufus, old friend. I goofed.

Rufus was a veteran, so we buried him in Forest Lawn Cemetery with a three-gun salute. Someone in uniform played a recorded version of taps on a fake bugle. Thus, I became the best male tapper in our group and the worst male tapper in our group because I was the only male tapper in our group.

Rufus: R.I.P.—rest in peace. The original Latin says the same in the same order—requiescat in pace. Rufus was a great tapper and much better than I will ever be. But he was of short stature. Consequently, female audiences didn't seem to pay much attention to him (he told me this, and he told me he was self-conscious and not happy with his height). It was the other (taller) male dancer that usually got the attention during performance—namely me. Rufus had a good smile and a happy, outgoing disposition. I miss him, and so do the others.

My happy tapping continued for a while until Judy Grace got sick with mesothelioma. Her sad decline into the dust was similar to that of Frances and too terrible to recount. Judy died December 7, 2014.

The wake was held in Galveston at the Malloy and Son Funeral Home, where Glen supplied plenty of hors d'oeuvres and margaritas. Food and adult beverages at a wake—that was a nice touch, and of course, that was Judy's idea. Judy was always considerate of our needs even after death.

The coffin was closed because Judy did not want us to remember her as a shriveled-up mess like Frances or like She in the 1887 H. Rider Haggard novel. On the lid was a color bigger-than-life picture of Judy in her prime, which is the way she wished to be remembered and is actually the way I am picturing her right now as I write this.

Judy was a very good teacher, and I know why. Before her retirement, she taught occupational therapy at the University Texas Medical Branch, and she was also program director for occupational therapy at Galveston College and at San Jacinto College South. She loved the applause and the foot-stomping and the audience cheers and the standing ovations from those in our audiences who could still stand. But there was something slightly unusual about how she always referred to the members of the audience. I never heard her call them residents, or people or inmates or old folks or gomers. To her, they were always "patients." She famously remarked to me, "I love to see the patients happy!" "It really is a kick when you finally see a smile on the patient's face." The other famous quote I recall her saying was, "You are not much of a tapper, Bernie, but you make up for it with enthusiasm. Your smile is infectious, and the patients love it." A left-handed compliment to which I had no rejoinder because, after all, it was the truth. Here's another Judy quote: "Today, Bernie, you danced better than usual."

Judy never distributed notes and never used them in her lessons. Like Frances, she never called anyone out. Her style and creativity will be long remembered. Judy taught me the Charleston, and I am the only kid on my block who can do it complete with bee's knees and with black bottom. Bee's knees is right out of the roaring twenties. Standing with feet apart or together, both hands on both knees, bringing knees together as the hands change places to the opposite knees, then open the knees again, and the arms are crossed, again bring knees together and return hands to the same knees, and open knees again with the same hands on the same knees, and continue over and over. The effect on audiences is amazing! The effect on grandchildren is equally good. Black bottom is also a step from the 1920s referring to the black bottom of: _____ (Fill in the blank. Hint: We are not talking here about the muddy bottom of the Mississippi river. We are talking about another type of black bottom,)

Black Bottom

Step R, Step L, Touch R hand to floor (that took guts, but eventually it seemed natural), Touch L hand to floor, Slap R hip with R hand move R hip to R at the same time, Slap L hip with L hand, and move L hip to L at the same time. Point R forefinger up high. Point L forefinger up high. With Judy in front doing the demo, it only took five weeks for our group to get these steps right.

Here Is the Major Lesson Judy Taught Me

Judy wanted me to learn a move she called heel clicks. I was against it because when she did it as a demo, it looked way beyond my capabilities. Tap terms vary from studio to studio and from one neck of the woods to another. What Judy called heel clicks is also known as bells, which consists of (what else?) clicking the heels in the air. Al Gilbert calls this "First position demi-plie in the air," which is a good definition, I suppose, if you know what a demi-plie is, which I don't. One of my other teachers (Noula Varsos) thinks heel clicks are heel hits, where standing on both toes, you strike the inside of both heels together by twisting both feet together, a maneuver that does make a click. The way Judy said to do her version was, "Lift your right leg to the side, jump up and bring your left leg to click heels together in the air. (This is neat, real neat!) Land on left leg with knees slightly bent. In all jumps, make sure you take off and land with a slightly bent knee. Look straight ahead and keep smiling." After less than 20 minutes, lo and behold, I could do this quite well, and, boy, it was fun. In the Veterans' Day show at Madison Jobe, I did this several times while representing the United States Coast Guard. Judy's clicks made me look like a drunken sailor. I discovered if I jump up with both legs, the maneuver looks more celebratory than drunk. Both styles were done at the Veterans' Day show. The audience went wild with each jump and click.

So, what's the point of this story?

I pause for reply.

The point is not how to do heel clicks or the bell or demi-plie in the air or whatever you want to call it. The point is you can probably do a lot more than you think you can. My attitude would have limited my progress if Judy had not helped and encouraged me. Don't limit your progress by preconceived ideas of what you can do and cannot do. Attitude is key. Have an upbeat, optimistic outlook, for that will serve you best. The lesson caused me to write a poem:

> If you think you can, you can
> If you think you can't, you're right again
> For
> Whatever you think you can or can't
> Is what you can or can't

Failures Now Do Not Mean Failures Always

Let's say you have two or three times failed to recollect a particular passage sequence in a particular dance, or you have failed to do a particular step like the time step correctly six times in a row. Do not assume and do not imagine that you will forget that particular sequence in the dance on the next occasion that you dance or that at some time in the future, you won't be able to do that time step. It took me several months before I could actually ball-change. Rome wasn't built in a day—or two days. It took me 99 hours of instruction and over 220 hours of flying before I got my pilot's license, and it took many years of flying before I was a master of the aircraft, able to complete all required maneuvers without serious difficulty or without significant doubt about my safe performance or safe outcome.

Trust Yourself: You Are Better Than You Think

A dancer who says to himself: "I know perfectly well that I shall break down in the usual place; it's no use, I simply can't remember it." is doomed to forget, for this form of auto-suggestion is fatal. To imagine that you can't do a thing is to very often render oneself incapable of doing it, as discussed. Moreover, it is of no service to a dancer (or to anyone else) to will herself/himself to remember something he has assured herself/himself that she/he cannot remember. Thus, when the imagination is in conflict with the will, the imagination will usually win. I am not saying the will doesn't exist or that it is totally disabled. I am saying that under these self-imposed restrictions, the will to remember will function feebly or arbitrarily or not at all. There is a long and complicated explanation for this failing, but let me just illustrate it in action:

Any normal person can, without much difficulty, walk along a twelve-inch wide ten-foot-long plank placed on the ground. No particular balancing powers are required for such a feat. But if the same plank were projected over the edge of a cliff, not one person in twenty could walk it. Why? In the last case, the person fearing that he may fall imagines that he will do so—tells himself that he will and then believes what his imagination has told him. From that moment, his actual power to walk the plank will significantly degrade so much so that he may indeed obey the compulsion of the imagination and actually fall. P.S. Don't try this experiment to prove me right or wrong. It is too dangerous.

Bottom Line

It is evident that in training the memory, one must at the same time cultivate the confidence in one's own powers. Without self-confidence, very little can be accomplished in any sphere of endeavor. You can do anything within reason. Your music memory is much better than you think. Your dance memory is better than you think. Self-talk is powerful. Give yourself frequent laudatory self-talk. It's fun and good for you. Usually, self-praise stinks, but not when it is just you addressing yourself. Try it and see if it helps. Also, here is another piece of home-spun personal advice: Never say anything against yourself for two reasons: Others might believe you, and (more importantly) you might believe yourself.

Dance Memory

Neurologists know that there is no practical limit to the powers of human memory in general and musical and dance memory in particular. Many of our great pianists have a repertoire of two or three hundred pieces, included among which are four or five concertos, say, a dozen sonatas, several works of the dimensions of Schumann's *Faschingsschwank aus Wien*, two or three of Liszt's *Hungarian Rhapsodies*, and perhaps 60 or 70 compositions, each of which takes eight or ten minutes to perform. These humans acquire this enormous repertory without any particular strain, and though, of course, many of them are specially gifted, there is no reason why the average musician who takes his work seriously should not at least memorize 50 works. Long ago, I set out to memorize poems. One a week or one every two weeks was my goal. Each night I spent 30 minutes going over the poem of the week. Now I can recite verbatim over 500 poems. Don't get me started. It sounds almost impossible, but after a while, committing to memory became second nature. There is no reason that with due diligent application that you won't be able to master 50 or more tap routines.

The Silver Stars Fall Apart

Because of dropouts and illnesses and boredom and who knows what else, the Silver Star Tappers were reduced to three. Judy Moody tried to teach, but she had had no experience as a teacher. She is an excellent tapper, but not a teacher. We tried watching the instructional videos made by Frances. They were of poor technical quality and manque. We tried working on some of the commercially available tap videos, including advanced *Tap Pups* with Vici Gruble Riodan. The lessons were watered down probably to appeal to a larger audience. The same thing is happening in books where authors don't present complex characters or deal with difficult philosophical ideas. *Tap Pups* does not deal with deep, complex art forms in tap dancing, probably to please a larger section of the public and, by that, sell more instructional DVDs. Sad to say, for the same commercial reason, most American films have descended to the level of TV melodrama and are now just part of the humdrum spectator culture of little real intellectual or humanistic value.

The End of the Silver Stars

So, we three, Judy Moody, Ester, and I, decided to disband the Silver Stars. Some costumes were donated to the Tappers of League City. Most of the costumes came to me and have been wonderful for the visiting grandchildren to play dress-up. What to do with the several thousand dollars in the bank was a difficult question. We decided to vote to decide what to do with the money. Ester said she agreed with the idea of voting, but she was not going to vote. Judy said the same. That left me with the only vote, and I decided Judy should get the money as payment for her work as teacher. Ester: "How come it's the man who always makes the decisions. Some of that money should have come to me."

I looked Ester straight in the eye, smiled my Master of Ceremony smile, and said, "Serves you right for not voting. Next time think twice before you disenfranchise yourself."

Judy and I then joined the tap group at Bay Area Senior Center (now renamed The Bay Area Community Center). Performances will remain in limbo until the Delta variant gets straightened out.

Noula Varsos is the teacher, and we are practicing multiple complex dances choreographed for the group by her. The idea is for every tapper to do the same thing in unison as an entrainment. It's fun, and we are getting back in shape mentally, physically, and spiritually. Someday, after the pandemic settles down, we will be ready to do shows. But for now, it is practice, practice, practice. Noula does do call-outs, and I personally am grateful for that. She is correcting my bad habits and has my interest at heart. There are two problems, of course: Unlearning the bad habit and learning the good habit. In one of Noula's dances, *All That Jazz*, I get to kick with the ladies in a chorus line. How many men get to do that? It's thrilling!

Noula introduced me to counting. This may help some people keep track of what's what in what part of the dance, but I rather doubt that real tap pros count when they are performing. Frances never counted, nor did Judy, and it is a rare event that I ever count when I am performing jazz or classical piano. Counting may be a learning tool. It is too new and too early for me to judge. Counting could count (pun intended) as an association tool that facilitates memory in some people, but I doubt it. In piano playing, for me, counting off the rhythm is a waste of time and tends to adversely affect the musical quality that I am trying to project.

Pandemic Blues

In general, there are lots of negatives about a pandemic, including the fact that so many people have lost their lives. Here in Texas, according to the Texas Medical Society, as of November 10, 2021, it is 70,766 dead. In the U.S.A., over 700,000 dead! Those are not just data points. Those are dead people who had friends, husbands, wives, children, brothers, sisters, relatives, and so forth. Since school started, there have been over 23,000 kids sick with Covid and 64 deaths! Tad, my son-in-law, says they are doing triage in Nashville because they lack enough machines to keep sick people alive. Thus, Americans are dying for lack of supplies. Who would ever have thought such a thing could happen here!

By the way, death is a bad thing. It spoils your week-end.

Pandemic Benefits

But there are some pluses, and one of those is the pause in activity that gives us time to think. And that, friends, is what we are about to do right now—pause and think. Pause and think about what was learned from our tap experiences. Some of these items may apply to your situation, and some may not. Read and decide. The lessons here described are thrown out in no particular order of importance. Later in the narrative, you will receive tips and tidbits that will help your memory in general and your tap memory in particular. And you will learn some brain science to help you better understand your brain and help you protect and preserve it. My method is one of improvised conjecture, a way of searching and not finding. There is no particular solution in mind for you or for me, but rather a love of inquiry and speculation for its own sake that often gives something to build on. Questions are more important than answers, especially the questions you ask yourself. Ideas are more important than lessons, especially the ideas you yourself develop.

OK? Let's start.

Dive in.

Talking Points and Topics

Teachers

My tap career spans over three decades, and during that time, I have had eight teachers. Three major teachers and five minor teachers. Frances, Judy, and Noula, the majors you already read about. Others taught me during the 2018 and 2019 Space City International Tap Dance Festivals sponsored by the Kennedy Dance Studio.

One teacher, a young, heavily tattooed woman, said during the break, "God, I'm horny. What say during lunch we go to a motel? If I don't get laid today, I'm going to go crazy."

"I can't help with the sex problem, but I do appreciate your teaching, and I am learning lots."

That afternoon, her lesson in musical theatre continued unabated. She was a good teacher, and that day I learned to tap to *Don't Rain on my Parade* from *Funny Girl*.

Another woman, a very famous tapper with a national and international reputation (I know her name, but I am not going to tell you), whose two books on Tap Dancing I had read, handled the class as if we were marine recruits at basic training. When she didn't like what a student was doing or not doing, she shouted, "Get out of my class!" By the time the hour was up, of the original 30+ students, there were only three of us left—two kids and me. During one practice step, she came up next to me, tapping, and whispered in my right ear, "You are a phony and a fake! We are doing a seven-count riff, and you are doing only five! You're lucky you're an old man. Otherwise, I would make you leave." My reply: "Thanks for the courtesy. I am doing my best and will work on the seven-count riffs at home."

In my opinion, this teacher's cruelty was unnecessary and probably reflected an ego defect on her part. As for me, I have such a big ego that stuff like that washes off my shoulders like rainwater. But some of the kids may have taken her criticisms seriously, and that may have damaged their egos and impaired their tap careers. It certainly damaged their fun.

Reader, if this so sad situation happens to you, change teacher or change studio. Do anything and everything to get away from toxic teachers and toxic people. Learning tap is hard enough without having to deal with the likes of them.

At Kennedy Dance Studio, there were two famous sisters from Columbia University who did jazz tap to a class of more than 80 students (I stopped counting at 80 because warm-up started). Imagine the thunderous sounds we made! All in rhythm! Technically, these teachers were great tappers but way above the level of any student in the class. So, I learned nothing, and I think most of the other students didn't learn much either. These teachers were more into showing off than they were into teaching. Which brings us to an important point: How would you like to have Ty Cobb as your batting instructor? Or Julia Childs as your cooking instructor? Their standards are so high, with them, you can't win. Select your teacher with as much care as you would select your lawyer or doctor or your spouse. Get someone you can relate to directly and who relates to you on your level. The teachers you have and their adoption tried, grapple them to thy soul with hoops of steel!

Know what you want out of tap and act accordingly. My aim was to have fun and develop some reasonable tap techniques appropriate to my age, station, and physical capabilities. Deal realistically with reality, or reality may deal realistically with you and sometimes rather harshly.

Performance

Among other things, tap is primarily a performance art. You should perform anytime and anywhere you can. Don't worry about what people think, and don't worry about making mistakes or looking foolish. Nervousness is just a precious waste, so don't get nervous. After you tap hundreds of times before audiences large and small, there is no way you will be nervous. You will be a native to the dances and to the manner born.

Tap on Cruise Ships

Ethel, my wife, and I love to cruise. On each and every cruise, there is a passenger show, and you can bet I do my thing. Several times on the Queen Mary 2 crossing the north Atlantic, I did solo taps to *Tea for Two,* and twice I did a nice charleston tap called *Doris.* One time on a cruise to Bergen, in the North Sea, I did a hustle tap. Of course, I made mistakes, especially in the charleston tap. I got off the beat, but the audience clapped me back on the beat and had a good laugh doing it. A life making mistakes is not only more honorable but more useful than a life doing nothing. The only person who knew about the mistakes was me, and I am very forgiving of myself, just as forgiving as the audience. The audience heard the off beats, but they didn't think there were mistakes. They thought it was part of the show. Afterward, a nice Japanese passenger told me, "That was a clever ploy of yours to get the audience to participate the way they did. I am crisscrossing but would like to social dance with you. But understand no sex. I am married. My husband stayed in London."

She was an excellent social dancer and obviously had taken lessons. Why she talked about sex, I don't know. It must have been on her mind. Some men think a woman is available if she asks them to dance. Not me. I am just flattered—no, that is not the right word—I am honored to have been asked. Some women just love to dance and want to dance with a man they think is a good dancer. She (the married Japanese woman) probably had been around enough to know it was important to make her position very clear from the get-go.

We did a nice rhumba and foxtrot together while Ethel watched.

On each voyage, the audience packed the place for the passenger show and cheered and clapped and stomped. Each time, I got a nice prize (prizes on the Wind Star were the best), including a certificate stating that I was the star of the show. Some evenings, when I entered the upper-class dining room (for example, Queens Grill on Queen Mary 2), there were resounding cheers. It is a rare event that any upper-class passenger performs in the passenger show. For one brief moment, I was a celebrity not just in the hallways and elevators but also in the first-class dining room. But how come no one asked for my autograph? I guess they didn't wish to disturb my dinner or theirs.

Where to Practice

Finding a place to practice on a cruise ship can be a problem. They stopped me from tapping in the gym on Queen Mary 2 because the tap noise was disturbing the afternoon nap of the German passengers in the suite below.

On Queen Mary 2, the best place to practice was the nightclub, which, except for the cleaning crew, is empty during the day. On other ships, I usually use the top deck, which is always nice wood and usually windswept and vacant. If there are any hardy souls there, I tell them I intend to tap, and they have always given their assent. Music is not a problem because the music is on my iPhone and the only one who hears it through my headphones is me. Expect, after about ten minutes, a small audience to gather, and of course, I acknowledge their presence with a smile and nod and continue practice. There will be time afterward to receive compliments and answer the usual questions: "How long have you been tapping? Where did you learn?" And from women of a certain age, "I used to tap as a child and wanted to go back to it sometime, but never did."

Some of us are tapping for the fun, and some of us are tapping for the adulation of the crowd, and most of us are tapping for both. Nothing like it! Make sure you get your share, and don't let silly shyness interfere with your fun and happiness. People care about entertainment. They enjoy watching the performer more than they care about perfection in the performance. They love bravery—the bravery of an amateur tapper with enough courage to hit the stage.

"Glory is fleeting, but obscurity is forever."
—Thomas Moore

Approach to Learning

Before jumping in. Look over your dance assignment and think about it for at least 15 minutes. Look for patterns. Try to visualize how you would work through the different steps. Talk to yourself about it. Point out interesting features. Discover what parts may need special application and attention and what parts are easy. Look for repeats. Try to link and associate the new material with things you already know. In my view, most students just dive in and lose the important step of actually thinking and focusing on the task and planning their attack.

Not convinced? Try this exercise:

Time yourself on this. You should finish in less than five minutes. To do the exercise, you will need a blank sheet of paper. Get your blank paper and then follow the directions exactly.

0. Read everything before you do anything.
1. Write your name in the upper right corner of the paper.
2. Print NAME under your name.
3. Draw a circle on the upper left side of the paper.
4. Draw a triangle in the circle.
5. In the middle of the page, calculate 43 times 956.
6. Make a large Q with a question mark in the right lower corner of the paper.
7. Draw a rectangle around your answer in item 6.
8. If you have carefully followed the instructions write "I have followed the instructions" at the bottom and sign your name.
9. Now that you have finished reading everything, you have done everything as directed in the first sentence (item 0), which was to read

everything before you do anything. Now don't do anything. Just place the blank sheet of paper back where it came from.

Ha ha ha.

At Rice University, where Doctor Patten taught the course *Mental Gymnastics*, most of the students set right to work and did not read everything before starting. The demonstration proved to them and perhaps proved to you that there is a tendency not to follow directions. And there is a tendency to just plunge in. Telling students that fact would not have been as effective as showing them. More than that: People see things more clearly when it is directly applied to them.

Performance Secret

The secret of good performance is feeling and understanding the music and the style and having a complete, firm memory of all of the steps of the dance you're doing and if dancing with a group. working well with the others. All that takes time, energy, and focus. The main thing, as I see it, is persistence. There is an old Irish proverb that states: "It's the holding that counts." If you can force your heart, nerve, and sinew to serve your turn when there is nothing in them other than the will that says to them, hold on—more power to you!

Dancing, in the opinion of many scientists, is the best way to fitness, better than running, swimming, gym, yoga, T'ai Chi Ch'uan, or walking. It is the engagement of the mind as well as the body, the emotional as well as the technical. For me, it is a skill in all senses of the word and one which has often given me an unmatchable natural "high." You agree?

On a basic level, tap is a better way to stay fit and more enjoyable than the gym. Tap does not rely on machines or weights. Tap is less laborious and gives results earlier. Work in a gym often will not produce results for weeks no matter what exercises are done. Whereas, I can feel increased muscle tone when I wake up the day after tap class. And, the gym is in a kind of public place where people are looking at you, how you do with weights and so forth, making appearances matter. In tap class, such considerations are way down the list.

Tap is open to almost everybody. All you really need is an ear for rhythm, two feet, and shoes that make a sound when they hit the floor. A ballet dancer is usually washed up after age 40. An Olympic star is usually washed up before age 30. But some tap dancers who start at 50+ and beyond (like yours truly) are still going strong. Example: Gene Kelly is still good at 80. All you need is two feet and tap shoes and the willpower that says go on.

No, change that. That is not quite right. Two feet are not needed. Peg Leg Bates dances on a single leg. Watch him on film and be mesmerized by what a single sound can do. The rhythms he creates are awe-inspiring, and he is a great success despite his disability. With one leg, he taps better than I do with two. Evan Ruggiero—same story. He also has one leg missing. But despite that, he can produce a rhythm that charms and impresses those who watch. Evan has a number of "pegs" that he uses to make different thumps on the floor while the other leg carries out the more complex tasks of using heels and toes. Evan and Peg Leg have great skill and a dance style all their own. More power to them!

Patience Counts

Be patient with yourself and your progress. It took me six months (believe it or not) to do shuffle ball change quickly and correctly. It took me many hours of instruction before I passed my airplane pilot's license flight and written exam. A younger student mastered the aircraft in half that time. So, what! Both of us can legally fly an airplane and carry passengers. Persistence and patience—that's the ticket.

The section on tap memory to follow will give some suggestions on how to develop your tap memory in less time with fewer tears. Meanwhile, some tips on practice.

Practice

Always warm up and cool down. Warm-up limbers the joints, muscles, ligaments, and tendons and thereby helps prevent injury. Detailed studies prove the dancers who get the best results are those who rest in between workouts. The exercise is to develop skills and strength and technique and so forth, and the rest is to help your body build tissue, strengthen muscles, and repair damage. Rest is just as important as exercise. Dancers who are overly enthusiastic and overwork are, according to recent studies, the dancers who suffer the most downtime and the highest number of serious injuries. If during practice you feel you are pushing yourself, stop and rest, recover your strength and energy and then, and only then, go back to what you were doing. Never push yourself hard. That's for Olympic athletes and not for the likes of you. Exercising to the point of exhaustion is a no-no. Do you want to get a heart attack or a stroke? Go easy. Practice should be fun, and if it is not fun, you need to make adjustments to make it fun.

Tap Dancing as a Sport

Tap dancing is not as dangerous a sport as much as boxing or football. But it can be risky and potentially harmful. There is in the leaps and lifts the chance of injury to the back and knees. And a fall is never far away. Falls in tap are the single most important fear in our tap group, and I don't blame them. Examination of the surface that we will tap on is my duty before the show begins, and I alert the group to what to expect and manage my tapping accordingly. We have to know in advance what carefree moves are safe and can be accomplished on a slippery floor, or a floor hard, or soft, or wet, or sticky, or sloping, or uneven. Be prepared!

Floors

Dancers need a wooden floor or a tap mat that actually gives a little, though the dancer is unaware of the give. Uneven floors, slanted stages, floors with small cracks where stage pieces are put together can be a problem.

Dancing on cement is probably a no-no, and it will not only injure your taps, but it may also injure your body. Knees are especially prone to injury from working on cement and hard surfaces. My high school track coach, Doc (Sidney) Elstein, bless his heart, never let us practice our running on cement or hard road surfaces or even cinder track. We trained on grass, and I believe that is the reason my knees are still OK.

It might be worth your while to look on YouTube or the internet for the black and white movies of the Nicholas Brothers or the Berry Brothers to see how far they pushed their bodies. They performed risky extreme physical moves for the sake of their art. That generation danced on surfaces that would not be countenances today in ways that now seem unfair to the body. Professional tappers require tremendous fitness and energy and (it has to be said) not a little youth. Those in their twenties in the chorus dances at Radio City Music Hall are fiercely rehearsed because it is this precision that makes an audience cheer the show and the Radio City Music Hall Rockettes to the rafters.

Distribute Practice

When practicing, you should remember the distributive rule. Multiple studies show you learn best when you distribute your learning over time with spaced intervals between tasks. In other words, do not cram. The major study that demonstrated the distributive rule comes from England. When they switched to zip codes, the British divided workers into two groups matched for age and sex. Group one was given 40 hours of touch typing, and group two had one hour of touch typing every week for 40 weeks. The group that had their learning distributed over time did much, much better on objective tests of typing speed and accuracy. It is not clear why distributing a memory task and a learned skill and not cramming is so effective. The current theory is that sleep consolidates memory (there exists lots of evidence this is so), and sleeping between lessons helps fix the memory.

Here's the way to think of it. The brain is like a muscle. Exercise helps make it stronger, and rest helps it recover from the exercise to build new tissue strength. The brain and muscle work best when not overworked, and they will work best when worked at intervals with adequate rest in between.

What does this mean for tappers? Which will be more effective learning for most students: One hour of intensive work on a single day or fifteen minutes of work on four consecutive days?

If you answered the 15 minutes over four days, pat yourself on the back because that is correct.

Mental Review

Mental review is almost as good as actual practice, and there is no need to put on tap shoes. You also can do your review work in street shoes, if you like, and profit almost as much. The goal should be to have a complete memory of the dance and each and every step in the correct order, done in the right manner at the right time for the right, artistic reasons with the correct arm styling and correct handling of props like the cane and hat. To help you reach that goal, you might want to know some things about the brain and how it works. Knowing about the brain might help you develop a tap program to suit your needs.

The Human Brain

Our brains weigh about three pounds, which for a 150-pound person is two percent of body mass. And yet, the brain uses at least 20 percent of total body energy and blood flow. Each brain has over 100 billion neurons, which are the actual brain cells. Each brain cell has structural helper cells and other cells to assist in nerve cell function. That brings the total number of cells in your head to about one trillion. There is a similar number of nervous system cells in the other parts of the nervous system (brain stem, spinal cord, peripheral nerves). So, there are about two trillion nerve cells in your body right now. That big number is nothing to sneeze at.

In olden days, it was thought once you were born, the number of brain cells did not increase and may have actually declined as you got older. You simply used what you were born with, and if those cells died through age or injury or drugs or whatnot, that was that.

Modern scientific studies show the brain can continue to produce new cells even late in life. That fact has been proven by scans and by autopsy results in volunteers who had special radioactive labels inserted into their spinal fluid before death. Thus, we are absolutely sure the brain, like the liver, skin, bone, and other body tissues, can, under the proper circumstances, regenerate and make new nerve cells. Human embryos make new neurons at an astounding average rate of over 5,000 per second during the 40 weeks of gestation. Yes, per second! That is not a misprint. Children up to about age two make new neurons almost as fast. Their brains are also busy making connections with other neurons, and such connections are called synapses. In just one cubic millimeter, there are in the human cerebral cortex over one billion synapses! Old folks also make new neurons but only at about 900 to 1,500 a day. Old folks also make synapses by doing things, and they lose synapses by not doing things. Use it or lose it. Neurons that fire together, wire together.

This massive collection of cells and synapses makes for a very complex organ, probably the most complex thing in the known universe. Some neurologists, myself included, think the brain is so complex that it will never be able to fully understand itself. But we try.

Neuroplasticity

Overwhelming evidence that is relevant and adequate proves that directed mental effort can favorably modify the structure and function of the human brain. This idea is called the principle of neuroplasticity, an important term that recently surfaced in newspapers, magazines, and on National Public Radio. Why not memorize the definition now so when the word shows up again, you know what idea is in reference? If you can work it in at the next dinner party, you will look smart.

Definition: A neuroplastic is a nervous system tissue that can modify itself to suit the needs it is called upon to fill.

In most cases, the neuroplastic is modality-specific. Therefore, it is not enough to decide you want a better brain. You have to decide what you want a better brain for. That is what specifically you want your brain to do for you. For instance, you can't wake up in the morning and decide you want a better memory. That is a wonderful wish, but it is too general and too non-specific to be of much practical use to you or your brain. You have to decide you want a better brain for a reason, usually a specific purpose such as "I want to memorize tap routines and dances more accurately in less time. Or you may wish to recite poetry better or play *Rhapsody in Blue* on the piano or learn French, Latin, or touch-typing. What's your bag? Sit back and think about this and actually develop your personal plan for self-fulfillment and development. Make it specific and concrete and put a timeline on it. Example: "By this time next month, I will know how to do the shim sham shimmy automatically from memory without much thinking about it in words."

The Ultimate Goal is Automaticity and Not Thinking in Words

Thinking in words and narrations about sequences as well as verbal labels will be discussed as tools to help you get initial control of your dance project. But the long-term goal is to do the tap dance automatically without use of verbal props. You want to be able to dance without much conscious thought, just as you can tie your shoes without much thinking or ride a bike. The idea of non-verbal thought puzzles some people when it shouldn't. Most of our thinking is non-verbal. Do you think about how you walk or climb stairs? Do you think Jackie Robinson has time to actually think about hitting that ball as it comes speeding toward him at 93 miles an hour? Most of what he does is non-verbal. It has to be non-verbal because there isn't enough time to think. And if he hits that ball, he will be just as surprised as the fans. Dame Margot Fonteyn asked Fred Astaire why he was renowned for practicing incessantly, demanding perfection in his work.

His reply was he practiced and rehearsed the technique so much so that when he came to film it, he didn't have to think how to do it and could get on with the business of performance.

How about Not Thinking in Words

For the last few years, I have been trying to train myself not to think in words. You might think that is a bad idea for a writer. But I don't know. It has advantages. If I don't let the words in, the stuff just flows in me, more or less quickly. I fix nothing. I let it go. Through lack of attaching myself to words, my thoughts remain nebulous most of the time. They stretch when vague, making unusual and pleasant shapes (sometimes in vivid colors, purples and greens mainly) and then are swallowed up: I forget them almost immediately. Thus, they can't haunt me. Albert Einstein repeatedly affirmed that he doesn't think in words, and his books indicate his main thoughts are images and pictures. Several scientific articles are about the visually mediated thinking of this great scientist. Isadora Duncan famously said, "If I could say it in words, I wouldn't have to dance it." She is thus admitting while dancing, she is not thinking in words.

Grey Lines with Black, Blue, and Yellow (c. 1923) by Georgia O'Keeffe is an evocative abstraction, recalling the interior of a flower and other forms like the vulva. Hailed by many as the "mother of modernism," O'Keeffe once said, "I found I could say things with colors and shapes that I couldn't say any other way—things I had no words for."

Stephen P. Hinshaw, Professor of Psychology, University of California, Berkeley, says in his course *Origins of the Human Mind* (The Teaching Company, 2010) that this kind of vague non-verbal thinking probably is the fundamental modern innovative force in both the arts and in the sciences.

I know I am fluent in French because I don't think of any English words when I am in France. The French just comes out spontaneously. Ditto when I read Camus in French. The French gives the meaning and the message, and there is no need for me to translate into English. That is the kind of spontaneity I aim for in my tap dancing. As yet, I have not reached the automatic stage. Words and narrative cues still help my performances, still help in memorizing the steps and sequences.

The Physical Basis of All Learning

Yes, our nerve cells and synapses are not fixed but can change depending on experience and need. This fantastic property is the basis for all learning. The plastic ability of the brain is responsible for multiple brain functions and skills useful in our everyday lives, including pattern recognition, visualization, narrative, language, naming and placing labels, and, of course, memory. More about these things and how they can help our tap dancing will be coming up soon. Meanwhile, back to neurogenesis, the making of new nerve cells.

Why Is Neurogenesis Important, and How Does All This Relate to Tap?

How well the brain produces new cells and how we can enhance production may solve age-related memory decline and perhaps even prevent dementia, including Alzheimer's disease. Thus, the goal of modern medical science is to find the best ways to enhance neurogenesis.

Unfortunately, studies on human neurogenesis are rather limited. Much of what is known comes from experiments on animals. Here is what we know so far as it relates to humans:

1.   Drug therapy does not work. No vitamin or supplement, or special diet has been shown to improve neurogenesis. The benefits touted on the internet are not real, but the profits from those who make those things and the profits that go to those who sell them are real.

2.   Gene therapy does not work. Genes inserted into the memory areas of animal brains increased the number of nerve cells, but no improvement is produced in performance or intelligence, or memory. In fact, the new neurons soon die before they have any lasting impact on function. Why they die is not known. The new cells do have trouble connecting with other cells forming synapses, and their failure to have synapses may activate a brain-specific destruction.

3.   The major finding in animal studies is and was and will always be that exercise triggers neurogenesis and that exercise has lasting effects on

animal intelligence. Young mice and old mice were put through exercise routines like running on a wheel. Aerobic exercise not only induces new neurons but also produces an important chemical called brain-derived neurotrophic factor (BDNF), a protein that plays a key role in nerve cell health. BDNF helps nerve cells survive and grow. Think of BDNF as a fertilizer for the brain, like a fertilizer for plants. Exercise also, in these animal studies, made the liver produce important chemicals for nerve growth and health (called Gpld1). The effect of exercise is not trivial. Exercised mice have triple the new neurons in their hippocampus (one of the memory centers) compared to mice who did not exercise. These exercise-induced brain cells form synapses and improve performance and memory. Therefore, exercise is key to brain health.

4. Conclusion: Right now, there is no substitute for exercise for neurogenesis. That is the current state of the art. Exercise is the only known effective tool to increase nerve cells and performance. Exercise is the proven adjuvant to brain health. The major mechanism appears to be exercise-induced production of brain-derived neurotrophic factor. Why and how exercise causes the production of BDNF is not known.

5. It is not clear from human studies what kind of exercise works best and how much is enough. Until such questions are resolved by detailed

studies, the current recommendation is 120 to 150 minutes of moderate aerobic exercise a week. A week—not a day. Moderation in all things, including exercise. Do not over-exercise. Anything that gets the heart rate up is good for the body and what is good for the body is good for the brain.

6. Therefore, there is every reason to believe that a consistent program of tap dancing will help develop new nerve cells and should improve mental and physical performance, strength, and endurance. I am sure it comes as no surprise to you tappers out there that the studies of humans who exercise regularly also show a significant improvement in mood. Every time I put on my tap shoes, I get happier. No kidding. It's well established that regular exercise improves mental outlook. And, researchers found from the data of the Health and Retirement Study, an ongoing project involving about 18,000 middle-aged and older adults, that exercise programs were highly correlated with people having developed a purpose in life, defined as "having goals and aims that give direction and meaning." (Reference: Journal of Behavioral Medicine, April 23, 2021.) Why exercise correlates with a purpose in life is not clear. Perhaps the people who have a purpose to start with are the ones who exercise. Perhaps exercise itself changes brain chemistry such that a purpose develops. Perhaps both

those two things are true. Detailed studies of runners show that running increases endorphins and DOPA, chemicals that make us feel happy. Probably tap dancing does the same, but we don't know that for sure, and it is not clear how such chemicals would produce a purpose in life.

7. Caution: Avoid the hype. Exercise is good. No question about it. But it just decreases the chances of stroke, heart attack, dementia, and so forth. It is not a panacea. You can exercise 24/7 on a thread mill, and there still will be no guarantee that you won't get demented or have a heart attack or a stroke. We are talking about probabilities here. By reasonable moderate exercise, you will most likely decrease the probability of dementia and vascular disease, nothing more. Your tap dance is an addition to, not a substitute, for the other things that will help your health, such as good nutrition, good social relations, a calm philosophical, optimistic outlook on life, and an environment free of air pollution, free of personal stress, and free of hazards.

Good genes and good luck will also help. Make sure you select your parents with great care and always carry a rabbit foot or potato (potato if you are Irish) for good luck.

"Potato I have."

Says Leopold Bloom, in James Joyce's *Ulysses*, as, before leaving his Dublin home, he feels his pocket for this Irish good luck charm, the potato, inherited from his mother.

Human Memory

A good memory is nice and often necessary for successful tap performance. Let's get to know how it works and how to use it. First, the definition:

Memory is a complex brain function that is time, modality, brain state, emotion, and lesion localization dependent.

Memory definition by division:

Human memory involves:

1. Time-dependent processes
2. Is modality-specific
3. Depends on the state of the brain at the time of learning
4. Is often influenced and even motivated by emotional needs
5. Can be lesion localization dependent.

General Psychological Research on Memory: Classic Studies

Current knowledge of memory relies heavily on the findings of classic studies by Ebbinghaus and by Bartlett.

Hermann Ebbinghaus was the pioneer, so we'll start with him.

Long ago in Paris during the spring of a year, a young German (or was he Austrian?)—no matter—was standing at one of those bookstalls by the Seine, the river that runs through that fair city.

There and then, he picked up a book, the name of which is not recorded in his autobiography, and he read something. What he read is also lost to history. But at that moment, that man had a sudden flash of inspiration—an idea that changed the course of human history, an insight that has significantly changed many lives for the better and that we hope will soon change your life for the better. Properly applied, the insights will improve your tap memory and performance.

A Brief History of the Dawn of the Scientific Study of Human Memory

The idea was to study human memory scientifically. Yes! Scientifically!

And to a scientist of that era (especially a German or Austrian scientist), the word "scientifically" meant quantitatively. By quantitatively, that man meant reducing memory to numbers by essentially measuring what was memorized and measuring what was forgotten, and (more importantly) measuring when, why, and how it was forgotten. "Measurement began our might," said the Irish poet William Butler Yeats. And he was right. All scientists believe if you can't measure something, you can't study it all that well. Numbers and direct measurements—very important in giving us insight into the nature of nature, the nature of reality. Business people know if you can't measure something, you can't manage it. The government understands this principle, and that is why it often issues figures about employment, unemployment, inflation, pandemic deaths, teenage suicides, climate change, and so forth.

Ebbinghaus, One of the Fathers of Modern Scientific Memory Research

The man at the Paris bookstall was Hermann Ebbing-haus (1850–1909), a doctor of philosophy and a genius. Hermann promptly returned home from Paris, kissed his wife, and then locked himself in his upstairs study to work on the complexities of human memory.

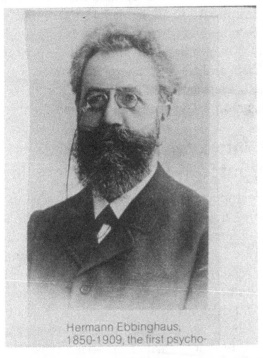

Hermann Ebbinghaus,
1850-1909, the first psycho-

Hermann Ebbinghaus, the first psychologist to study memory experimen-tally. He invented nonsense syllables, which he regarded as uniformly un-associated. Most textbooks will tell you he got his idea of studying memory quantitatively from reading Gustav Fechner's book Elements of Psychophys-ics, and that was the book he found at the Paris bookstall. But if that were true, why did Hermann not mention that in his autobiography?

Hermann Ebbinghaus' Experiments

Using himself as the one and only subject for his experiments, Hermann Ebbinghaus devised 2,300 three-letter nonsense syllables for measuring memory. In a typical experiment, he would pick the nonsense syllables at random from a hat, review a list of 16 of these until he could recall them perfectly in two faultless executions aloud, and then retest himself at various time intervals recording the results. All in all, he had 420 lists, and each took about 45 minutes to memorize. He estimated he did at least 14,000 repetitions. While the time spent memorizing the lists and the number of repetitions were closely correlated, Hermann found the number of repetitions done was more important than the time spent.

Key Point: Number of Repetitions Is More Important to Memory Than Time Spent

There are important physiologic reasons why this is true, reasons we now know to be true, reasons that do not concern us here. In fact, a Nobel prize in Medicine was awarded for the discovery of the brain mechanisms that underlie repetition as the major mechanism of learning. Just remember this: Neurons that fire together, wire together. And then, it follows as the night the day, neurons that are wired together will fire together. Key ideas like these are often more easily memorized as verse:

Neurons that fire together
Wire together
Neurons that wire together
Fire together

The lesson is clear: Repetition counts. Repetition is an important part of learning and memory. Without repetition, very little learning takes place. Without repetition, very little learning can take place. We repeat: Repetition is important. I repeat: Without repetition, there will be little learning. One-step learning is possible but usually for only simple tasks. Large projects and important memory tasks require repetition. Was there ever anyone who could memorize *Casey at the Bat*, all 52 lines, without repeating the poem many times? You don't remember, but it took many repetitions before you could tie your shoelaces, or ride a bike, or could walk instead of crawl.

To memorize just one performance dance will require lots of repetition, and you will hear your tap teacher say, "one more time, one more time, and one more time" many times. You, as a tapper, must realize there will be an initial period of extended practice and dedicated repetition before you can achieve something that is pleasing to the ear. And with that practice must come the visual look added, which is a whole other aspect! Tap is not easy and requires an intelligence in the ear as well as in the feet. And tap dance is cerebral, and because it is cerebral, it will be, and it is extremely satisfying to the soul when it is mastered.

Why Repetition Makes Memories

Repetition causes neuronal networks to fire together and wire together, and once they do, they tend to be more easily fired together, the very process that underlies human memory. When you start your memory work in earnest, you will recognize how repetition starts to make recall easier and easier until, at last, recall is automatic.

Repetition is so important that you will find that things are often repeated in this book. No harm in that, and actually, the repeats will help you remember. But hear this! Stupid parrotlike repetition, especially when you are not mindful of what you are repeating, does away with concentration. Our repetitions must be patterned and organized. Repetitions must be mindful and focused. Rote memory = bad. Repeat out loud: Rote memory is bad. All repetition to be effective must be mindful. The brain gets bored fast. When you find your interest or your attention diminishing, stop and rest or do something different. Rest periods are a good time to talk with and socialize with your tap friends. The rest periods should refresh your brain and will help you memorize tap routines.

Repetition Has a Dark Side

As we learned, when you repeat something over and over, the nerve cells in the brain form new connections. This is how you learn things and how you form new habits. The more you repeat something, the stronger the connections between the nerve cell networks. But there is a problem. You may have noticed that once you have developed a habit, it is really difficult to change it. That is because the connections in the brain that form the habit have been formed by lots of repetitions over time. To unlearn a habit or to replace it with a new one, you have to repeat the new habit many, many times so that the brain changes the old connections and forms new ones. In tap practice, for instance, if we repeat the passage steps many times incorrectly, the brain will actually learn the incorrect form of the music, and there will be a devil of a time correcting the mistakes and getting things right. The key point here is that in repetition of anything with a view to remembering, make sure that you are repeating as carefully as possible, avoiding any and all errors. This applies to memorizing music, songs, poems, history, math, or anything. The important part of repetition is to repeat correctly and not repeat incorrectly. Each time you do a correct repetition, you are writing a protected spot in your brain. Each time you do an incorrect repetition, you are also writing a protected spot in your brain, a spot that will be difficult to erase or change without lots of work. Practicing errors will not give you the results you want or need. Therefore: Always practice right! And never practice wrong! But this raises the question: How do we know what is right and what is wrong? The main answer is to consult the written notes and choreography. The score and the notes are your friend. Review them frequently to make sure you are practicing right and not practicing wrong. When I review, I am usually shocked by how much I missed, what mistakes I made, and what sections and steps I completely omitted. The notes focus my attention on what is wrong, and they tell me what needs work. When there are no notes, some students make a video of the dance and review at home from the video. Whatever works for you, do.

* * *

OK, Hermann Locked Himself in His Room and Repeated Nonsense Words—So What?

So what?

No way, so what. You should be thinking: Wow!

Think about it! Locking yourself in your study for three periods each day 10-11 a.m., 11-12 a.m., and 6-8 p.m. for over four years and memorizing masses of meaningless lists. That's dedication, dedication to science. And mind you, all this must have been tedious and boring. Tenaciousness is considered by some as a particularly Teutonic trait. If that were true, then Hermann's work would be a great example. He carried on, despite the fact that his work must have been boring.

Must have been boring?

YeeeAhhh!

What are we talking about? It was boring. Hermann says so in his famous book published at Leipzig in 1885, *Über das Gedächtnis (Memory, A Contribution to Experimental Psychology)*.

Hermann, in confidential moments, admits his brain loses its "freshness" after 20 minutes and becomes bored. When each test required longer periods of concentration, say—¾ of an hour, he admits, "and toward the end of this time exhaustion, headache, and other symptoms were often felt which have complicated the conditions of the test."

One wonders how many headaches were generated to learn that lesson.

What lesson?

Lesson: The human brain fatigues quickly. The human brain quickly loses its focus, becomes bored, and begins to shut down. If you are tired or bored or sick, forget about memory work until you are ready and eager.

At-TEN-shun!

Failing to focus is one of the biggest things that interferes with memory. You can't remember something to which you didn't pay attention. Think about that. It could be the reason you are not doing well in tap lessons or in science class or in everything else that you are not doing well. You are mentally absent instead of mindfully present. What's the treatment for that?

Answer: Pay attention! Also, take frequent breaks to refresh your brain. A break every 15 minutes is good. During the break, focus away from what you are doing. Focus onto something different so as to refresh your brain.

* * *

Get It, or You Will Forget It

You have to get it. Or you'll forget it. But this idea begs the question. The more important question is—How do we get it? That's the key question: How do we train ourselves to pay enough attention in the first place to get the items we want to remember into our memories?

Lesson: Boredom prevents and often kills memory.

The best bet is **AVOID BOREDOM**: Do a small amount of mental work at a time, take frequent breaks, and vary the subject matter, work on things that are fun and that interest you—about those techniques, more later,

Meanwhile, let's talk about what our hero Hermann accomplished despite the boredom and despite the headaches he endured.

Despite the headaches, the dull, dreary, mind-numbing humdrum, Hermann persisted. He exercised willpower, something we all can use to advantage in our mental exercises and in our tap practice. In fact, this is something I need to work on to improve. Even during class, I find my mind wandering. Often when I should be following along on the next step, I am thinking of the stock market, or what Ethel might make for dinner, or why my right knee is hurting.

And my distraction is not particular to myself. It afflicts most humans. A famous study at Harvard Law school had students press a button whenever they discovered that their attention had wandered and they were thinking of something other than the law lecture. At any moment in time, an average of more than 30 percent of students were not paying attention! And those are highly selected, very capable students. You can tell a Harvard man, but you can't tell him much.

The distractions can be legion. Learning to forget the distractions and learning how to concentrate attention will be one of the most important things you will ever learn. Don't believe me that your mind wanders? Try this experiment. Relax in a chair and focus your attention on one thing, say an image of a coke bottle. Within ten seconds, if you are an average American, another thought will pop into your head. Yes, our ability to concentrate is that bad.

Back to our hero.

After he got an individual list memorized (as was mentioned), he retested himself at timed intervals and recorded what he recalled and recorded what he did not recall. Along the way, he proved human memory is a complex process that is time, modality, emotion, and state-dependent. Remember? Sound familiar? Some, not much, of the complexity will be covered later in this book. But it might be useful for you at this time to rememorize the definition. Memorize it either as a statement:

Memory is a complex brain function that is time, modality, emotion, brain state, and brain lesion localization dependent.

Or memorize the definition by its divisions:

Memory is a complex brain function that is dependent on:
1. Time
2. Modality
3. Emotion
4. Brain State
5. Brain lesion location

Each of these items is important and is explained in detail in my other book *Making Mental Might: How to Look Ten Times Smarter Than You Are.* The brain lesion thing is interesting, and neurologists love stuff like that. Neurologists know there are special sections and areas of the brain which when injured, prevent verbal memory. Other sections, when injured, prevent visual memory, or taste memory, or smell memory. The brain consists of a hierarchy of modules that have special modality-specific functions. And, yes, there are sections for particular types of memory for sounds, such as memory for a fire alarm or a ringing phone. Those patients who have damage in those special areas understand speech and can talk quite well, but they are deaf and blind to the meaning of the non-verbal sounds like a bird call or mountain lion roar, or a door bell. There are people who have sections of their brain-injured who can speak and understand words but can't repeat anything you say to them (known to neurologists as a disconnection syndrome called conduction aphasia wherein the speech detection system is disconnected from the speech production system due to a lesion in a deep white matter tract in the left hemisphere known as the arcuate fasciculus). There are patients who can write their name or anything you dictate but can't read what they just wrote. That syndrome is known in neurology circles as dyslexia without agraphia and is due to a lesion in the posterior corpus callosum and the right visual cortex. The patient can write anything but can't read anything, even what they have just written. Fascinating right? Neurologists love this stuff. Me too. But it is not important for you at this time.

What is important is knowing how time, modality, emotion, and brain state affect memory. Knowing how those items work and what role they play in memory will help you get through any memory task.

Confusion in Trying to Remember Similar Lists

Hermann found if he worked on one list after another, the first tended to interfere with accurate recall of the second, and the second tended to interfere with accurate recall of the first. In psychological circles, this phenomenon is known as proactive and retroactive inhibition. In tap, this problem shows up when two similar dances are studied back to back. The more they resemble each other, the greater the problem in getting each straight. Hermann's conclusions were based on non-associated meaningless letter combinations. If there is meaning and association, the proactive and retroactive inhibitions tend to disappear, and the confusions become easier to manage. So, make your associations and labels and narratives to serve your purposes and help keep things right. If two dances are very similar and you are having trouble keeping which is which, then avoid the problem by working on only one of those dances.

Serial Position Effects

The other problem Hermann found with items in a series (that is, a list) was that the probability of recall relates to the position of the item in the list with the items at the beginning and at the end recalled best and the middle items often not remembered as well. In psychological circles, this phenomenon is called the serial position effect. It is well documented and plays a role in remembering any series of items, any list, any dance, and in playing classical piano pieces from memory. You will also notice the serial position effect when you go to the movies. In general, you will remember the beginning and the end of the movie better than you remember the middle. Don't believe me? Test yourself after you have read a book or a newspaper article. Usually, the beginning and end are recalled much better than the middle.

The same holds for me with the tap dances. Usually, with me, the end is remembered best, and then the beginning is remembered next best, and then the middle is recalled least well. The remedy is to put more energy, attention, and repetition on the middle of the dance than you ordinarily would. If I concentrate on the middle sections and review them more, the serial position effect tends to decrease but doesn't always go away entirely.

The Famous Forgetting Curve

Despite the complexity, our man Hermann proved memory, under certain experimental conditions, can be measured almost exactly. His most important discovery, and the one for which he is very well known in psychological circles, was the "forgetting curve" that relates the amount of forgetting to the passage of time.

Memories Fade with Time

Yes, time! Time is the real enemy of mankind, and time is the real enemy of memory because human memory degrades with the passage of time. The forgetting curve proved that fact now and forever. As time goes by, you remember less and less. Is there any doubt about the adverse effect of the passage of time on memory? You will know and adequately perform a tap dance many times only to find several weeks, months, or years later you have forgotten most of what you knew so well. Do not despair. This is normal, and you will find that reminding yourself of what you knew will often bring the memory back in far less time and with much less effort than it took you to memorize the dance in the first place.

Recent research proves forgetting is not just a passive process. The brain actually and actively erases what you do not use. The brain pays attention to what is often recalled to consciousness and tends to forget what is not often called to consciousness. Use it or lose it. Furthermore, it is very interesting that if you review only part of a dance that you have forgotten and neglect to review the parts you knew so well, you will tend to forget the parts you knew so well in favor of the other stuff you are concentrating on. In psychological circles, this phenomenon is called **Retention Fatigue**. If you just work on the new material and neglect what you know well, the brain assumes the stuff you know so well isn't important and tends to erase the material. The lesson here is to briefly review everything, not just the problem parts. I always go over the parts I think I know so well before I start to work on the parts I have forgotten. That bypasses the Retention Fatigue problem by calling the brain's attention to the old material and alerting the brain that those previously learned items are also to be remembered and not neglected.

The Brain Knows Nothing

Remember, the brain knows nothing. The brain assumes what is frequently presented to the consciousness is important and encodes it in the memory. The brain assumes what is not frequently presented is not important and tends to forget it. So, the paradox will be that you learn the material you didn't know and have forgotten the material you knew so well. The treatment is to briefly review the material you know. I do this at the start of my learning session. Because I know it already, review time is short, usually less than five minutes. This is an important concept. If you don't understand it or are unclear about it, please re-read the above paragraphs. You may want to make a narrative to help you remember about retention fatigue. How about: "If I don't review what I know, I may lose it due to retention fatigue." The narrative memory tool you dream up yourself will work better than anything I or someone else dreams up for you.

Recency Effects

There is also a difference in remote versus recently learned material. Dances learned during the Frances era are almost completely forgotten. Dances during the Judy era are less forgotten, and dances under current review with Noula are even less forgotten. You already knew that, right? It is called the recency effect. Review of material just prior to performance will help the performance due to the recency effect.

Emotions also play a role in the quality and quantity of memory. The dances I like are more easily recalled and more easily memorized than the ones I don't like. Trying to memorize a dance I hate is such an uphill battle that I learned long ago not to do.

Tip for school kids: A short review before you are actually tested will work wonders, especially on multiple-choice or short-answer tests. Space your learning and reviews out over a long period of time, but just before the test, do a fast look-see.

Lesson: Review time is never wasted. Review what you want to remember and forget the rest

Back to Hermann and the forgetting curve:

The forgetting curve remains one of the eternal verities about human memory performance. There are other eternal verities about human memory, which we will cover, but that one, the forgetting curve, is among the most important. Never ever forget the forgetting curve. Another way of saying the same thing: Always remember the forgetting curve.

Not incidentally, there is also a learning curve. It is exponential, just like the forgetting curve, with the sharpest increase in learning occurring on the first day. After that, the learning curve levels out much like the forgetting curve.

Efficient Learning

Maximum efficient memory for items in terms of time invested occurs when review time equals the original learning time. For a one-hour lecture, the most efficient review will be one hour. For a one-hour tap class, the most efficient learning will occur with one hour of review. Sure, more study will get more results, but here we are talking about the best and most efficient use of your time. We are talking about the best memory reward for the amount of time invested in review. And remember, the best review will be spaced out, taking advantage of the distributive rule. Therefore, the best way to review a one-hour class lesson each week, assuming you don't work on weekends, would be one hour of review divided into review sessions lasting 12 minutes each over a five-day period (60 / 5 = 12).

Active Learning in the Community

Learn to work and play well with others. Lots of data is available now, but here we list for your consideration the big six items:

1. Growing consensus holds that humans learn best when they are active (not passive).
2. When people are mentally engaged and not distracted.
3. When material to be learned is meaningful and not disjointed.
4. When learning occurs in a socially interactive context.
5. When learning is iterative and not merely repetitive.
6. And (this point is key) when learning is fun!
   Reference: Science, October 1, 2021, vol 374, issue 6563, page 27.

Time-Dependent Processes in Human Memory

There are two important time-dependent phenomena in human memory that Hermann studied quantitatively:

A. Forgetting and

B. Encoding

Let's look at these items one at a time. Forgetting first.

A. Forgetting is the default mode of human memory

In a certain sense, the news about the forgetting curve ain't good: The default mode in human memory, as mentioned, is to forget and to forget quickly.

In the list of 16 nonsense words (like WUX, CAZ, ZOL, BAZ, etc.), for instance, which Hermann had memorized perfectly, only eight could be correctly recalled one hour later, and only five could be recalled after two days. Thus, overly learned material that had been recalled perfectly twice had slipped out of the memory at the rate of about one percent per minute for the first hour. After two days, the rate of loss tends to settle down until a relatively constant level of retained information is reached two weeks later. Hence, if you can recall only a fraction of what you have read in the introduction to this book or a fraction of what happened to you two hours ago, don't fret or worry. Your memory performance is quite normal. Perfectly recalled material two weeks later, if encoded without associations, will no longer be perfectly recalled. In fact, you will be lucky to recall more than 30 percent of what you previously knew perfectly. That is the nature of our memory problem. We have to learn to live with it, and we have to learn how to get around it. Question: Can you think of a way around this problem? Hint: Would getting to tap class and reviewing what you covered and learned previously help?

Memory, Thy Name Is Frailty

If you have played a piano piece perfectly twice from memory, say *Für Elise* by Beethoven, don't be surprised if you forgot half of it the next day. And don't be hard on yourself if, without review, two weeks later, you forgot 70% of it. That's the norm: 30% correct recall after two weeks and 70% forgotten. Expect the same thing if you recited from memory Lincoln's *Gettysburg Address* perfectly twice. You will forget almost half of it the next day, and one week later, you will recall less than 30 or 40%. However, despair not: A brief review will work wonders in bringing back the previously learned material if you have learned it well and were able to reproduce it perfectly at least two times. With each review session, the time to relearn the material will shorten. If you don't believe me, try learning your next tap performance and retest yourself at intervals to see how much you remember and how much you forget. Since most of us have too high a rating of our own performances, it is a good idea to record your repetitions and review them. You will be surprised by how bad they look and how much you hesitate, and how much you have forgotten. That's good. How can you improve if you don't know what needs improvement? The other advantage of recording is that you will actually prove to yourself that you are making progress if you are, in fact, making progress.

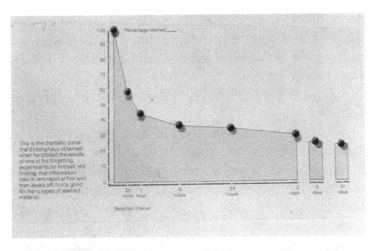

The forgetting curve for unassociated perfectly learned three-letter items.
Note the dramatic drop in retained material after just one hour. Within
24 hours, over 60% is lost forever.

But what's the deal? How come we forget so easily? How come we have to work to remember?

Here's the answer:

We need to forget almost everything.

There are important reasons that our brains are biased to forget: Most of the stuff we come into contact with in our everyday lives just ain't that useful or important or that memorable. Just think of what a nightmare life would be if you remembered every little detail of every little thing that happened every little moment.

"To remember everything is a form of madness."

—Irish proverb

That's what we need. Right? We want to remember what we want to remember, like a Mozart piece, *Für Elise*, the spouse's birthday, the electric bill, and so forth, and we don't want to remember what we don't want to remember. We want to remember the French word for cat if we want to buy a cat in France or say the word correctly in French class tomorrow.

Goal #1: Forget trivia; Remember the important stuff.

That begs the question. What is important? The answer to what is important is what is personally important to you: What interests you and what you want to remember. No one can tell you what is important. You have to decide for yourself. Your brain usually doesn't know what is important. You have to tell it. The brain assumes something you do often or think about often is probably important, and that is why repetition and habit fix memories.

Remember What Is Important

It's nice to remember the important stuff like your spouse's birthday, when the mortgage needs to be paid, when the garbage gets picked up, to bring the math homework back to school, where you parked the car at the airport, that the door is locked, stove off, cat fed, and so forth. A good memory can come in handy in many ways.

The trick is to remember the things that are important and forget what is not important. The techniques discussed in the pages coming up will allow you to do both (remember and forget) and give you control over your memory that you (perhaps) never thought possible. If the tap dances are important, you will have a better chance of remembering them. If you don't care about a particular dance, if you consider it unimportant, you won't remember it.

Bartlett

Bartlett (1932) became interested in the kinds of information that people remember rather than the number of trials needed to memorize that information. Instead of asking people to learn lists of nonsense syllables, Bartlett used meaningful stimuli such as words, objects, pictures, meaningless inkblots, and stories and measured the extent to which the memory of the items changed over time. For instance, his method of repeated reproduction required participants to read an unusual story from folktales or myths and later recall the story after various periods of time. He found recall was often characterized by omissions, simplifications, and transformations, thus proving that memory is often vague and incomplete. Alas. Human memory, for the most part, is terrible and not a reproduction at all but rather a reconstruction wherein participants' errors changed the story into more familiar and conventional forms. When individuals did not actually remember part of the story, they tended to fill in things as if they did. And after they reconstructed the memory, many of the subjects believed their reconstruction more than they believed the original material when represented to them. Lawyers know all this all too well, and that is why they want to get depositions as soon as possible and also want to "woodshed" witnesses and correlate what one witness says with what the others say. This defective witness idea is a gigantic problem in law enforcement. My father was the District Attorney of Queens. He would put on a trench coat and stand in the line-up and was often picked out by the witnesses as the perp. One year, the DA's office had a black clerk. He was often IDed as the rapist in multiple line-ups! The truth was that women were simply unable to identify the rapist, but they thought they could. Most men with black skin are not rapists and are, like this law clerk, decent law-abiding citizens. I shudder to think how many men, black, white, yellow, or whatnot, have been falsely accused of rape and are now suffering in prison because of misidentifications. The most grotesque creatures (like these false witnesses) arise because nature generates them, like toadstools. They exist because they can't help it. We must beware of them.

Even eye witness accounts were unreliable, and yet the eyewitnesses seemed overly confident about what was, in fact, defective recall of the event. A robust psychological literature has demonstrated that testifying witnesses are, even at baseline, pretty bad at memory recollection, confirming Sir Frederic's observations. Asking someone to recall details after years have passed is even more precarious, like trying to ask a toddler to do calculus.

All in all, this real-life research paints a dreary picture of the capabilities of human memory, and the main takeaway message from Sir Frederic C. Bartlett's overly long and boring book (entitled *A Study in Experimental and Social Psychology*) is that our memories are quite defective and unreliable. The results caution us to verify what we think we know and retest and prove we know it. Be advised to review, repeat, and practice whatever you really want to know by heart.

If you think Sir Frederic's book is not boring, you haven't read it. But, you know, we always profit from reading. In my view, the interesting aspect of *A Study in Experimental and Social Psychology* is the detailed explanations by the subjects on how each as an individual approached the memory problems. Basically, the people divide into two groups. One group used visual methods of encoding the memory, and the other used verbal methods. The visual group would make a mental image of what was to be remembered, and then at recall time, they would summon the image to consciousness and read the to-be-remembered items from the image. The images were often vague, and this group made many errors of recall putting stuff in that was not there in the first place and omitting things that were there. Really interesting and discouraging was how sure they were recalling things correctly. In the visual group, there was overconfidence in their memory, and they were usually cock sure they knew what was what when they didn't.

By contrast, the verbal group did much better at recall, especially the stories and even the pictured items. They approached the memory task by labeling things and making narrative links from one item to another. The verbal group looked at the memory problem as an exercise in logic and tried to encode information in a logical sequence. The verbal group's very effective tool was verbal chunking. They divided the to-be-recalled items into associated groups, and they remembered by recalling the group name and then reeled in the items from that group. This group was very keen on pattern recognition and labeling the pattern to help subsequent recall.

When a label was clear, they used it. For instance, a circle in a hexagon. But even with the inkblots where there was no pattern, they would imagine a pattern and use the imagined pattern for recall. For instance: "This inkblot is nothing, but I can imagine it looks like a duck turned on its side and walking on one foot, and that relates to the next ink blot that might, with a stretch of imagination, look like a fox after the duck." In contrast to the visual group, these people who used mainly verbal memory tools were hesitant and unsure of their recall. Their evaluation of their performance underestimated their accuracy. Sir Frederic had no explanation for the results, nor do I. Was it something they had for breakfast that hurt their sangfroid? Why did visual memory not work as well as narration, chunking, labeling, and imagined pattern recognitions? We don't know. But it is a fact that verbal clues and cues and chunking and narration are effective in promoting accurate recall of anything.

Short Notes as a Chunking Tool

Judy Grace taught me about short notes as a memory aid. First, you memorize the dance. Then you reduce the dance to a series of short notes that will tend to trigger the memory. For example, here are my short notes for Vecchio. These are hardly interpretable if you are not already familiar with the dance. But if you are familiar with the dance, a brief review just prior to show time will usually help and sometimes will work wonders. Notice I am also using place memory by reminding myself where page one ends and that will shift my attention and my (usually) weak visual memory to page two, where we find step five, which is shuffles. Place memory in humans is strong, much stronger than time memory. Some people can actually picture the choreography notes on a page and can read the notes from their mental picture. If you can do this, more power to you. My images are there but too vague for direct readout. The vague image, however, and its position on the page does help me remember what's what.

Intro—Toe Heels and Snaps

1. Shim-sham
2. Vine with essence
3. Do-si-do
4. Flaps with coaster steps
   End Page One
   Page Two
5. Shuffles
6. Riff
7. Buffaloes
8. Timestep

How about you? Want to test yourself? Try this picture and make a mental image of it by studying the picture for three minutes by the clock. One hour later, recall the image and the items and see how you did. Write out your answer so that you do not fool yourself into thinking you remembered more than you did.

Next, look at the picture for three minutes, name the items, and group them into chunks of related or associated items. The chunks have no existence in nature. You are the one that assigns the items to groups. A cigarette, for instance, doesn't know it belongs to the smoking group and can be associated with an ashtray. We can associate cigarette with ashtray because we know the ashtray is a good place to drop cigarette ashes. Get it? You make the chunks with your imagination. After one hour, test yourself to find out what, if anything, you recall. Write down what you recall so you don't fool yourself into thinking you did better than you actually did.

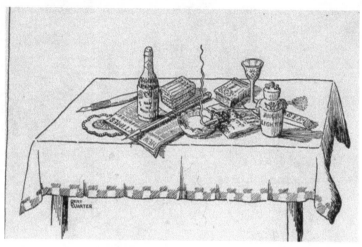

Here's What Happened When I Tested Myself

Visual—Unable to see any image in my mind's eye and therefore unable to recall anything except I know there is a table with a table cloth. Thus, my visual recall memory is zero items remembered using a mental picture.

Verbal Organization and Narrative: There is a smoking group with cigarette, pack, ashtray, lighter fluid, and matches. There is a writing group with pencil, pen, newspaper, book, and eraser. There is a drinking group with bottle, glass, and doily. So, I need to remember three groups; smoking, writing, and drinking. When recall time occurs, I will think of each group in turn and then try to remember the individual items in each group.

Recall after one hour. Lit cigarette with smoke, cigarette pack, ashtray, and lighter fluid, but I forgot the matches. I got newspaper, book, pen, pencil, and eraser. I got glass, bottle, and doily. So, 12 of 13 items were recalled. That's 93% recall when the psychological studies expect only 50% recall. Although I used mainly verbal tools and chunking, I did have a vague sense of seeing the table and the items bunched on the table but was not able to actually identify or read out any item from my vague mental image. One thing I did notice, though, was each time I recalled an item to consciousness using words, there appeared in my mind's eye a more or less vague image of the item in the picture with the correct location of the item to the other things in the picture. For instance, when wine glass came to consciousness, lo and behold, there was a vague image of the glass summoned to mind by the name *wine glass*, and I think I almost can see the wine glass positioned among the matches, book, and lighter fluid. Not only that—I think I see (vaguely but there) the shadow cast by the glass and the interesting design on the glass that I had not noticed before.

How did you do? Can you see the tremendous advantages of putting labels on your tap steps and putting the steps into chunks and also the benefit of narrating the sequence of the labels to yourself? Did you apply any organizing principle to your memory task? Organizing items into groups and then reading out the groups can help your tap memory. For example, in one dance I do, Tack Annie comes after steps one, five, and seven. Examine your performance. Note what helped you and note what did not help. If something helped, tell yourself what it was and see if you can figure out why it helped.

If you did not do this exercise, you missed out on proving to yourself whether verbal chunking or visual imaging or both will help you remember things. If you didn't do the exercise, shame on you. Who do you think you are fooling? But wait! All is not lost. The exercise will be here waiting for you whenever you wish to come back to it to give it a try.

Examples Applied to Tap

Most tappers use a number system to organize the sequence of tap steps. After the introduction, there will be step one followed by step two and then followed by _____ (guess). The number system is a well-learned part of our mental life, and the exact sequence of numbers is available as pegs on which to hang items to be remembered. We learned from the psychology research that our memories are frail and that forgetting is the default mode of the human brain. We can bypass this fault by association of the thing to be remembered with something we already know, or we can simply make up an association link. Let's say the introduction has finger snapping. How can we associate introduction with finger snapping? The best association is the one you make for yourself. An association I make for myself will work best for me but may not work as well for you. Here, I simply connect the introduction with finger-snapping by a narrative that says:

118

"This intro is a snap." The chunking tools that we use to follow will be the tap steps we have memorized, labeled, and practiced many times so that they can be reproduced almost automatically the way you automatically tie your shoelaces.

Usually, if we can correctly recall the first part of a given step that we have rehearsed several times, the other parts will quickly and automatically fall into place. The reason for this phenomenon is that the sequence of items or steps is linked and associated consciously or unconsciously in our minds. Associations, any kind of associations, will build memory. Usually, if you hear the first few words of the lyrics of a song, even one you have not heard for 50 years, you will be able to fill in most of the rest. Just hearing the music will remind me of the lyrics of songs from long ago. Unassociated memories are different. They are frail. No associations? Then expect the drop in memory exactly following the forgetting curve for the forgetting curve was derived by unassociated memory task of meaningless combinations of letters.

Making Associations Is Important

"Ideas developed simultaneously or in immediate succession in the same mind mutually reproduce each other, and do this with greater ease in the direction of the original succession and with a certainty proportional to the frequency with which they were together."
—Aristotle (384–322 BC)

When most of us hear someone say the letter A, we automatically think of the letter B because B comes after A, and we learned to make that associative link long ago

119

in a time out of mind. In the same way, we can, by narrative links, connect one tap step with another.

Let's work out on one of Noula's dances to see if we can apply what we know about memory in practice:

Vecchio

Since I don't know what Vecchio means, I looked it up. Vecchio is Italian for old. Why this dance is named Vecchio is not clear. A reason for the name would help our memory of the dance.

Intro: Center stage: Hold eight counts, four toe heels with four finger snaps in place, four slow toe-heel jazz box with four finger snaps.

Jump on right, point left

Jump on left, point right

Slide right to left foot, slide right to left—hold 7 ball change right (&8)

Method: Narrative—intro is a snap. Intro has three parts: Snaps, jumps, and slides with ball change. Snaps, jumps, slides. SJS. Multiple associations help the memory and are useful. The brain is not overburdened by application of multiple memory tools. Use as many memory tools as you need.

Repetition: Practice group of snaps, then jumps with points and slides. After doing this five times, this should come automatically. If you have trouble connecting snaps with the jumps, tell yourself, "After the last snap, I do jumps, first right then left."

Self-test: Do the entire intro from memory. Record your performance to make sure you did it right. Correct mistakes and omissions. When memory is firmly embedded, work on style, smile, and grace. Give snaps "that look." Soon you will do the introduction automatically without giving it much conscious thought. That is the desired effect.

What do you think comes logically after the introduction?

If you said *step one*, give yourself a pat on the back or take a break as a reward.

Step One—Label this as you please. Having a name attached to the step beside the number one will help association of step one with the intro. Example: "Intro goes to Shim sham bombershays with reverse." The steps follow but would be more easily recalled as just two chunking tools (Shim sham & bombershay—right and left.)

Right heel dig, brush step right

Left heel dig, brush step left

Right heel dig, brush step ball change

Right heel did brush step

Chunking: heel dig brush steps right-left-right ball change (no step), then right brush step

R L R b/c R

Play with this a little. Make your own narratives and associations. Expand or contract as you see fit. What you do as an individual tapper to get the dance into automaticity is more effective than anything I or anyone can suggest to you.

Bombershay to left (1& 2& 3& 4)

Shuffle ball change step right clap.

Analysis: Step one follows the intro. Step one divides into two parts, a part with shim sham and a part with bombershays. Then the two parts reverse. Note: If you had previously memorized shim sham and bomber-shay, you could use those names as chunking tools.

Memory work: You know the drill. Repetition. Narration. Self-test and so forth. Make a video of the intro followed by step one. Most of you out there are too lazy to do this, but those of you who do will be amazed at how well you do. As usual, correct mistakes and review. If you argue that the method takes too much time, I would argue that it will actually save lots of time because once and for all, you will have gotten the to-be-remembered steps in the memory.

OK, take a deep breath, and now using the memory tools you have just learned, memorize the first two steps from Al Gilbert's Training Aid #1157, Musicworks 42nd Street. Time yourself from start to finish. Consider it memorized when you can repeat it correctly twice:

STEP ONE

a. Eight flaps starting right entering (flap 2, 3, 4, 5, 6, 7, 8)

b. Flap R, shuffle L, ball change L-R twice and reverse. (Flap shuffle ball change ball change. Flap shuffle ball change ball change.)

c. Repeat a & b.

STEP TWO (facing front)

a. Stamp R, hold, ball change L-R, stamp L, hold, ball change R-L, step R, step L (stamp ball change stamp ball change, step step).

b. Brush R forward, hop L, step R forward and reverse, ball change R-L and repeat twice, turning right. (Brush hop step, brush hop step, ball change x three turning R.)

c. Step R to R, drag L to R, ball change R-L twice moving R and reverse. (Side ball change ball change, side ball change ball change.)

d. Repeat b of step one. (Flap shuffle ball change ball change. Flap shuffle ball change ball change.)

Check your work:

Give yourself a checkmark for the memory tools you used:

1. I did not just plunge in. Instead, I read and reread the steps and focused my attention on relationships and patterns for at least 15 minutes.

2. I used repetition to memorize the steps.

3. I tested myself to see if I got the step correct actually doing the steps.

4. I divided the task and worked on small parts at a time.

5. I used name, labels, words, and narrative tools—any, all, or any combination.

6. I recognized the patterns involved, such as step one has two parts that repeat, and step two has four parts, but the last part (d) is from step one, and I recognized there are two ball changes in step two c and d but only one ball change in step two a and b.

7. I talked to myself to remind my conscious mind where I was and what I was doing and what comes next. Watch out: The self-talk should not be a mental pep talk on how you are doing so well. The content of the talk should relate

to the content of the dance. Sometimes mental pep talks, such as "you are doing great," "you can do it," and "keep up the good work," don't help and will actually derail a performance. Beware pep talks. Pep talks can provoke just the opposite counter thought that you are kidding yourself and will ultimately fail, and they usually distract you from focusing on the task.

8. I felt a feeling of joy and accomplishment when I mastered these two steps from 42nd street.

9. I used personal imaginative associations to facilitate the memory of the sequence of steps.

10. More? You fill in and add what you used and did. Give yourself extra credit if you made a video to check your work.

Grade

Give yourself a passing grade (C+) if you used each of the following: Focused attention, repetition, pattern recognition, self-test, narration, and self-talk with verbal clues or cues or both.

Review Time

We covered time-dependent processes in memory. For tappers, there are two key points: Memory fades with time, and review reconstructs the memory. Human memory is modality-specific. If you want to learn tap dancing, studying Chinese won't help. "Plant bean, get bean." is an old Chinese proverb. Practice tap, get better at tap. Emotions are important in human life and play a role in your tap career and tap fun. Do the things you like and don't do what you don't like. You will perform better if you relate to the dance emotionally, as well as intellectually, as well as artistically. Current evolutionary science says the emotions play a major role in motivating humans to action. For example, fear motivates us to fight or flight. Love motivates us to mate. Depression motivates us to protect resources. Let your affection for the music and the dance motivate your learning.

The more pieces that you have memorized, the better equipped you will be to improvise a dance. Only one of my three teachers has had us improvise in class, probably for good reason. Most audiences prefer choreographed dances to improvised ones. But, and this is a big but, most of the tap books I have read emphasize the importance of devoting ten minutes a day at home to just putting on some music and developing your own tap dance to that music. The more dances in your repertoire, the easier this is and the better it looks. For some reason, the dances that I have invented for myself seem to play better before my family and friends than the dances I have learned in class. I am not sure why this is so, but I think it might mean that I put more of my soul into my own dances. Because I relate to the *Doris Tap* dance and its provocative lyrics and joyous Charleston steps, it is the dance I love to do during passenger shows on cruise ships.

Brain State and State-Dependent Learning

The state of the brain during learning is important because if the brain is not in the same state during the performance as it was during the learning, then the playback will be adversely affected. Astronauts who learn things in space have trouble remembering the same task on earth but quickly recall what they learned when back in space. Drunks who hide money while drunk may not remember where they hid the money until they get drunk again. In tap, brain state plays a role in rehearsal for performance. Working in front of the mirror in the studio is one thing but working in front of the audience without the mirror is another. Try to do rehearsals that closely simulate playback conditions without the mirror, and try to be dressed as you would be for the show. Other dancers should be spaced and positioned the way they will be positioned at showtime. In other words, try to simulate in rehearsal the situation that will exist during the actual performance.

Chunking Tools

We will soon cover the common tap chunking tools. These are as essential to tap as the scales, chords, meter, and rhythms are to playing the piano. These are as essential to tap as twinkle, inside turns, and balance steps are to waltz. Once tap chunks are learned, they will make memorizing any tap dance easier and faster. The chunking tools displayed here are the ones I know. Others can be found in Al Gilbert's wonderful tap dictionary *(Al Gil-*

bert's Tap Dictionary: Encyclopedia of Tap Terminology and Related Information, Stepping Tones, 1998)) or use actual tap flashcards that are available on the internet. Learning to do the chunks will be easy for some people and hard for others. But all will have to do some work because there are lots of these and many are complicated. In fact, they amazed me when I first met them because I never imagined there were so many things you could do with your legs and feet.

Toe-heel—two sounds

Step down with the toe and then drop the heel of the same foot. This can be done walking in any direction or in place or as a jazz box. Try walking forward with a series of toe-heel right, toe-heel left, toe-heel right, toe-heel left. Do this to music, and the overall effect will create a sense of accomplishment even if you are a beginning dancer.

Toe tap—one sound

Touch the top of the toe to the floor. This can be done in any direction, front, side, or back, but usually is behind the other foot, close to but not touching the other heel. A dig is heavy emphasis of the foot or toe or heel in any direction. Heel digs are usually is done in front.

Step—one sound

Step down on the ball of the foot with weight. Touch is the same without weight.

Stamp, stomp, slam—one sound

Stamp is stepping down with the whole foot with weight (also known as a flat tap). Stomp is the same with no weight. Slam is with emphasis with or without weight and is usually done with a straight leg.

Shuffle—two sounds

Brush forward with ball, then pull (back with a brush back). Do this in front of a teacher or a fellow tapper who knows what's what so you can get the proper sounds and speed.

Scuffle—two sounds

Hit forward with heel and then pull (brush back). Rhymes with shuffle and is almost the same but not quite.

Riff—two sounds

Brush and heel scuff in one motion as you extend your leg. A true riff has only two sounds.

Three count riff—three sounds

Riff followed by a heel drop on the other foot. Brush-scuff-heel. This is real cool once you can do it automatically.

Paradiddle—four sounds

Heel, spank, toe, heel. Frances tried to teach me this one. It isn't hard if you remember to start with the heel, and if you remember, it has four sounds. The word itself has four syllables. Frances worked long and hard with me to try to get this right, but so far, I can do it slowly, but I can't do it fast enough to use it in a dance. So, Frances would let me phony the paradiddle, and of course, no one noticed, and no one cared. Fake it until you make it.

Leap—one sound

Go from one foot to the other foot in any direction. A leap always has a change of weight from one foot to the other. Leap is my favorite because it has such great joy in movement. Put weight on one leg and then transfer the weight to the other. At the same time, I usually straighten the departed leg and put arms on a diagonal with the arm that is down is down on the leaped to side. This creates an iconic image, an iconic image of tap as iconic as corte is iconic for tango. At home, during improv, I do leaps right to left and repeat. This maneuver has not been tried in studios, but it really gives a great effect and is fun. Personally, I have always been in love with the freedom of expression that dance can give. I have not been too drawn to disciplined learning, although I do recognize the need for some structure. So far, all of my teachers have been "old school," and tap innovation has not been encouraged. That's expected because tap is pretty much old school.

Leap brings up the question of what to do with arms. My motto is "When in doubt, arms out" or second position at sides. Ballet or jazz arms are good, if and only if they relate to the particular tap dance. There are no set arm positions in tap, with the possible exception of opposition arms. Open arms and arms opened send a message of reception and friendship and happiness and accessibility. Closed arms, especially crossed arms in front in protective gesture, are off-putting. Arms fixed to the side or dangling down might be OK for *River Dance*, but tap is an American dance and should express American freedom with the freedom of American expression.

Jump—one sound

From bent knees, spring into the air from both feet and land on both feet. You can jump from any position on two feet to any other position on two feet. Pushing both arms up when in the air and folding them back when landed creates the visual expression of great joy. Try it and see.

Hop—one sound

Hop is a jump on one leg to land on the same leg. Bend the leg slightly, jump up and land on the same leg while smiling and adding arm styling. Seniors shy away from hop and do what they call "senior hop," wherein they merely quickly lift the heel on one side and then put it down. This takes less time and lets the seniors keep up with the music and the younger dancers. Most seniors I have seen make two sounds when they attempt a real hop, and that is wrong.

Heel scuff—one sound

Heel scuff is a brush you do with (what else?) your heel. Scuff the back of your heel against the floor as your leg extends to the front or side. My heel scuff looks like I am kicking a football, except my heel hits the floor in the process.

Heel drop—one sound

With your weight on your toe, drop your heel to the floor to make a sound. The heel drop sound tends to be lower-pitched and less loud than other sounds, and you have to use judgment to decide whether or not to turn up the amplitude. Some tap sounds are tricky to get right, and this is one of them. Tap sounds must be clear and pure.

Heel, heel hit, heel dig—one sound each

Heel just hits the floor with the back of the heel. Heel hit hits the back of the heel tap against the floor and lifts the foot after, whereas the heel dig hits the back of the heel tap against the floor with the heavy emphasis of more force and does not lift. Heel dig is really a heel made with emphasis.

Flap—two sounds

This is a key step and worth much practice to get it right. A flap is a brush and a step with the same foot. Very basic and very important. It can be done in any direction, but the usual is forward. A flap always takes weight ever so briefly. A slap is like a flap but is a brush touch with the same foot and does not take weight. Slap can be done in any direction. Flap and slap are always two sounds.

Cramproll—four sounds

Ugh! Into every tapper's life, a little rain must fall. Here we have what can be daunting if you don't keep organized. If you do keep organized, it will come easy. Cramproll is a series of steps and heel drops. You can cramproll in place or moving in any direction. Forward cramproll would be step right forward, step left forward, drop right heel, drop left heel. Thus, RLRL or step, step, heel drop, heel drop. Add a flat to the first step, and you get a five-count cramproll. For some reason (probably because right-left resembles walking), this step comes quite naturally to me. Others have trouble with it because, I think, they think too much about it, and that spoils the natural automatic nature of the step. It is like thinking of how you are breathing. Paying too much attention to this seemingly ordinary act can make you self-conscious and disturb the breathing. Thinking too much about tying your shoe may actually make it harder for you to get it done.

Ball change—two sounds

Step in any direction on the ball of the foot and then step on the other foot. This changes the weight from one foot to the other. Practice this forward, to the side, in back, and in place.

That concludes the steps considered basic. There are many more fun steps to learn. They have unusual names and sometimes many names for the same step. One of my favorites is waltz clog, which also carries the name Pat Rooney because he invented it. Waltz clog is my routine warm-up step. Cotton-eye Joe, a Frances favorite, is another warm-up I like. How about Broadway? Buffalo? Maxie Ford? Timestep? Timestep is so standardized now it has become a fossil, but it still serves a purpose in that it creates a benchmark for all learners going into the world of tap from children to adults. Because so much of dance is steeped in tradition, we are hard-pressed to change it, even if we could; we may as well try to rename Christmas.

There are so many steps and dances to learn and so little time. And tap not only has many steps. It also has many mansions, many forms. There's soft shoe, military tap, Irish tap (that had a revival in 1997 with *Riverdance* and *Lord of the Dance*). There's funk tap, which is mostly close to the floor, as performed by Savion Glover in the show *Bring in the Noise, Bring in the Funk*. And there is novelty tap, Latin tap, jazz tap, and eccentric tap (also called Legomania), a comedy style of tap with very loose stylized movements. Ray Bolger was a great exponent of eccentric tap (Ray was the scarecrow in *The Wizard of Oz*). You already read about Joy Nall and me, who did boogie-woogie tap to jitterbug 4/4 time as our signature duet. Honky tonk tap based on 2/4 or 4/4 and old-time ragtime and Dixieland were among Frances' favorites, and we enjoyed learning them and dancing them.

In fact, let's face it, tap dancing is an art form so deep and so varied no one will ever fully master it. But we tappers keep trying.

OK. That's it!

Here ends Mister Hollywood's Completely Nonessential Guide on Tap Dancing.

Vale—Farewell-Goodbye

All good things have to come to an end. And this little chapbook is no exception. Sorry about that. Try to hold back your tears while I explain that where you go from here is entirely up to you. You can acquire more knowledge and skill, or you can stay the same standing still, or you can fall back as you please. You are the master of your fate. You are the captain of your soul. Spend some time thinking about your future directions. Meanwhile, I sincerely wish you—

Happy tapping!

Your friend,

Mister (Tap) Hollywood

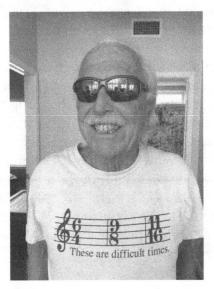

ADDENDUM: TAPPERS' TRUE TALES

The Magical Tap Shoes

By Lou Ann

One day there was a tap class at the Madison Jobe Senior Activity Center where I was the Director. It was the usual class that was held weekly, but this time I was walking through the class and did a couple of steps just to kind of join in for a few seconds, and quite frankly, I loved tap from the moment I put on tap shoes as a five-year-old. I was invited to join in the class, which I wanted to do but was a bit out of shape and practice, so feigned an excuse that I couldn't possibly dance that day because I didn't have the proper shoes. So, this spry, fit guy in the class piped up with sparkling eyes and asked what size I wore. I replied that I wore a ladies' size 11, thinking full well that there would be no shoes there that would possibly fit me.

He gleefully stated, "I've got an extra pair in the car that ought to fit you just about right." He quickly changed his shoes briefly and went out to the car to get his extra pair of tap shoes. I was then put right on the spot to put up or lose face. I had a feeling they were going to fit, and I was going to have to tap dance that morning. When he arrived with the shoes, he brought a pair of socks that were mostly clean, as I remember. So, I put on the socks and the shoes. The shoes were actually pretty perfectly broken in and were a perfect fit. It was almost as if the shoes were magical.

So, then, with no excuses now, I spent the rest of the class time tap dancing with the class and laughing and missing a few steps here and there but mostly just dancing and enjoying myself. I was happy that I remembered most of the basic steps. All the problems of the day vanished for the moments I had those shoes on. All I could think about was tapping to the music and laughing. I was facing a mountain of issues at the time, and those magical shoes made all those things that were weighing on my mind vanish for the time being.

Later, when the class was over, I reluctantly offered the shoes back to the gentleman. He replied, "No, just keep them with my blessings. I have several pairs." Those were the best fitting tap shoes I may have ever had on my feet and I truly coveted them. So, I was elated.

To me, that day and forever, those tap shoes were magical, and I kept them in my office to use again. I put them prominently on my bookshelves so that I could look at them and smile and remember the gifts I was given that day. I received the gift of laughter, the gift of letting go of my problems for a moment, the gift of joy, as they certainly brought joy into my life, the gift of being included, like being picked for the kickball team first, and the ultimate gift of love and generosity in the giving of the shoes themselves.

I kept that pair of shoes on that shelf until I retired from the center. I consider them more precious than diamonds, and they have a prominent place amongst my shoes so that I see them every day and remember the joy that they brought into my life.

And that spry guy who could dance so well who gave me those magical shoes and who was always so full of enthusiasm, spit, fire and vinegar was none other than the author of this book.

The ripples of a kind act spread far and wide and seemingly never end, somewhat like the ripples of water in a lake when a stone is thrown.

I was transformed that day to that five-year-old girl in the pretty black lace and gold satin recital costume, complete with net arm puffs, tap dancing to the tune of Chattanooga ChooChoo and somewhat surprised that almost 60 years later, I could still remember that first performance routine.

Thank you, Bernie!

* * *

Miss Scott's Story

I used to enjoy morning walks 'round the neighborhood, sometimes with friends and sometimes by myself with my dog.

I was looking into doing other activities, and I asked my friend, "Do you know if anything is going on at the Community Center?" She said, "I have heard things, but I have never been over there."

The next day I decided to go look for myself. It was a Wednesday. I spoke to the receptionist at the door, and she gave me an activity schedule with things to do; I thought I heard music coming from another room and wanted to know what was going on. I sat down and saw these tap dancers; I have always wanted to learn tap dancing but never had the opportunity. I waited until the class was over, and I asked if they had a beginner's class. I spoke to a lovely lady, and she asked me if I had taken tap lessons before, and I told her no. The only dancing I had done was at school, the dance was called The Highland Fling, and we got to wear our kilts. She asked me if I could come in the next week to see how it would go. She told me that the three steps most important in tap were a shuffle, a shuffle ball change, and a 'flap.

I was so excited to go back the next week. I was surprised to learn that I was not the only beginner in the class. It was so much fun. Some of the girls knew a lot more than just the beginners; We all stayed at the back of the class, and we watched the other girls with more experience. I learned to do a 'shuffle ball change and flap, it took me a while, but I was determined to learn.

The weeks turned into months, and we were starting to learn a dance called Hot Honey Rag. It was a thrill to get dressed up with colorful scarves and feathers in our hair. We had red lipstick on and big necklaces and silver earrings. We looked like "floozies" for five minutes. I probably was the worst in the class. I like doing crafts, and I volunteered to make the headpieces for the dance. One of the girls I tapped with was a Professor at the University of Houston, and she said we could practice in her classroom on a Sunday afternoon. It was great news to hear because I could go to tap on Wednesday and tap on a Sunday.

Every year the Community Centre had a craft day. They named it "Christmas in July." We were told that if we learned Hot Honey Rag, we could dance on the craft day. I didn't think I could do it. My teacher said, "it's not for another month," and you're getting better. I was determined to dance at that craft show, and as the saying goes, "fake it till you make it."

I practiced until my feet hurt. I was tapping in my sleep. That Sunday, we were at the U of H for several hours. I was so happy I had achieved Hot Honey Rag

When I went to my Wednesday class, I knew the whole dance; My teacher was impressed at how well I was doing. I told her I had been practicing a lot. She was curious, and it was then I told her I had a secret, and it was at the University of Houston practicing tap. I sometimes go to the Community Centre in Friendswood on a Friday, and I get to tap there too.

I have been tapping now for about seven years, and in that time, I have been to almost every class. It makes all my troubles go away, and I love every minute of it.

The thing I like best is going to the senior citizen homes. I love to make them happy with the dances I have learned. They love all the colorful outfits, and we always get a 'round of applause; I like to dance in the back because I have always been a bit shy, although I am getting better. The one thing I am not very good at is dancing and smiling at the same time. One of the dancers always tells me to SMILE.

Some people say, as you get older, your feet don't work the way they used to. I am not going to let that stop me; As long as I can move and my health is good, I will be tapping. When the good Lord decides to take me, you can bet your bottom dollar I will be dancing in heaven if I get there.

* * *

A Tap Story from Ms. TEXAS

I do not remember when I became interested in tap dance. But when I first saw people tap dancing, I realized that the human body is a fantastic instrument capable of making exciting, joyful sounds. When I was 55 years old, I was searching for another career. Instead, I found a tap class at the Bay Area Community center. Tap dance is very sophisticated and requires fast and flexible moves for me. I was hesitant to attend the tap class because I did not have any dance education or childhood dance experience. When I attended the first class without tap shoes, my teacher lent me used shoes, and I followed her dance. I did not recognize how fast one hour and thirty minutes passed. Tap dance gave me joy, energy, fulfillment, and strength. I was so excited that I could make tap noises with rhythm.

After the first class, I googled some basic tap steps and followed the YouTube instructors. I decided to buy used tap shoes from eBay and watched YouTube for basic tap steps almost every day. I also made my own tap board and practiced around 30 minutes three times a week. I also asked for tutoring from an experienced tap dancer from my group.

A few times a year, our group has been performing tap dances at nursing homes. I am an introvert and nervous in front of people, so when we had a performance, it was not easy to smile while remembering my steps. I wanted to improve my tap steps and my movement, so I searched for movies with tap dancing in it. I watched the tap dancers' facial expressions and the movement of their arms and legs. It made me more enthusiastic to dance, and since then, I have had an interest in old movies and musical movies.

One year after starting tap dance, I moved up to the intermediate-level group. This group performs more complicated steps and various dances. Even though I was afraid of speaking or performing in front of audiences, I desired to perform tap dances on the stage. I was nervous, but I decided to enjoy my tap dances with the mindset that even if I might make a mistake, I will just smile.

I met wonderful senior tap dancers, and they are good at tap dance, and my tap teacher guides me to dance better. Our group members always encourage each other and try to maintain their health and their strength from their passion for tap. It is beautiful to see their passion, especially as an aging group. When I look back on six years of tap dancing, I want to become a person who expresses myself through tap dance with passion. I am still learning how to make clear tap sounds and get a good balance. I hope I can keep tap dancing with more smiles while I'm still on this Earth.

* * *

My Dream of Dancing Was Always on My Mind

By Anne Miller Wannabe

Since I was a small child, tap dancing has held a special place in my life. My family's religion frowned on dancing, so dance was strictly taboo and not in the foreseeable future. My pursuit into the arts would be through music.

I began piano lessons at age five years old and continued taking lessons until I was ten. At ten years old, I lost interest and the lessons stopped because of lack of practicing.

My dream of dancing was always present in my mind, and I took advantage of any opportunity that came along to learn about dance.

During my elementary school days, there was a group of girls that would practice acrobatics such as tumbling, cartwheels, and hand stands at recess. Also, there were a few tap steps (flaps, ball changes) that were demonstrated by a friend that took tap dances.

As I started junior high school, some of the girls went to different junior highs, and dance was put on the back burner for a while.

Studying and school functions filled my life through high school, and the only dancing I participated in were school dances.

Fast forward to my adult life, which consisted of pursuing a college degree, getting married, and raising a family.

My friend, whom I met when she and I were room mothers for our children, wanted to start a dance studio. She had a strong background in dance since she had danced professionally and also had auditioned for the New York Rockettes. She did not make it because of the height requirements. She was not tall enough. She wanted to have an adult tap beginners' class and invited me to join. I told her I would love to join, but I had not had any formal dance lessons. She said not to worry, I would fit in just fine.

My first official tap class was at age 42 years old.

I also had started back to college after a twenty-year hiatus, so dance became my stress release from studying.

My original tap class was terminated after two years because of lack of interest. I was able to find another adult group and expanded my dance repertoire to include tap, ballet, jazz, clogging, Irish Hardshoe, and Irish soft-shoe.

Dance mainly tap was my stress release while obtaining my nursing degree at age 46 and my master's degree at age 56.

As I have progressed to my senior years, tap is the only dance I do. I danced with a senior group (Silver Star Tappers) until they disbanded and then joined the Bay Area Community Dance group. I still love every practice session and also entertaining seniors in nursing homes and senior events.

Tap is a form of exercise to music that has kept me fit, improved my agility, and increased my stamina as I have aged. If you have a love for music and dance and are in your senior years, I recommend tap dancing as a way o stay fit and enjoy life.

* * *

Bic's Story

I didn't put on a pair of tap shoes until I was an adult. During my childhood in Houston, Texas, I longed to dance, but good things come to those who wait.

The lower-middle-class family I grew up in had the necessities: a home purchased with the GI Bill, food, clothes, and sometimes adequate transportation. The six of us lived in a small three-bedroom home with one bathroom and no air conditioning. For several years, we did not own a television. Many of my clothes were hand-me-downs from cousins, and our car was usually an unreliable jalopy.

We did not have luxuries, particularly in the form of travel or outings to movies, concerts, the circus, the rodeo, or the Ice Capades – all fun things our classmates talked about. We were an academic family, and when we were not engrossed in homework, my siblings and I played board games and read books from the Bookmobile that stopped in a shopping center parking lot once a week during the summers. I learned to sew. Outside, we roller-skated on the sidewalk and rode our Dad-made bicycles.

What we did have was a great nuclear and extended family. However, neither side of the family was all that musically inclined. Our neighbor Frances, who eventually had six daughters, made sure they all had dancing lessons. Once, she took me along to well-known Hallie Pritchard's dance school near downtown to observe. It was a long drive to the studio with her growing family, and even if my parents had agreed to lessons, I would not have enjoyed that drive on a regular basis.

Frances and another family friend with daughters who danced invited us to their yearly recitals, which were free at the Music Hall in downtown Houston. I loved watching, but it saddened me that I could not participate. My dad said the dancers he had known as a child during the Depression were snobs. I suspect the real reason was that my parents did not find music and dance to be a priority when finances were stretched enough already. My brothers did get to play

Little League baseball through elementary school; it did not cost as much, and Mom found a way for the family members who needed braces on their teeth to have them!

In intermediate school physical education classes, I was hopelessly unathletic. The saving grace was the indoor unit on folk dancing and square dancing during the winter months. It was so much fun, especially if you had a great partner. As it was a girls' PE class, my partner was always a girl. My friend Debbie, blessed with more athleticism than me, was also a good dancer, and she was my partner in eighth grade. When we finished up for the season, the teacher suggested to Debbie and me that we sign up for drill team training when we chose our high school freshman year courses.

Surrounded by girls who had been dancing since they were toddlers, I had a lot to catch up on in drill training. To this day, I still take a long time to learn a new dance. At the end of the year, Debbie and I tried out for the drill team. Debbie made it, and I briefly became an alternate. To my mom's dismay, the performing uniform rentals were not cheap, but she purchased the fabric, and I sewed my own practice uniform and the dress and jacket we wore to school on game days. Three games into the football season, I earned a regular spot on the performance team. I did not know why the girl I replaced had left the team until a year later when she showed up at a football game with a baby in her arms. I gradually improved, becoming known for my high kicks and splits. Then I became vice president of the team my senior year.

In college, I once again faced my lack of athletic ability in a physical education class. Only 5 feet 2 at the time, I was horrible at basketball that first semester. Then I discovered a tapdancing class was to be offered in the spring semester. That's when I got my first tap shoes!

Only five young women were in a class taught by a kinesiology graduate student. Most of us had never tapped before, but within a few weeks, we were hard at work choreographing our own dances. I remember one classmate danced to Ringo Starr's "You're 16," and I made up a dance to Al Hirt's "Java." On April 1, we arrived at class, and the instructor told us the men's PE program coaches were considering adding a tap class for them, and they wanted to see our dances first. We were perplexed but started rehearsing for the impromptu performance. Then the instructor laughed and said, "April fool!"

After college, I finally had my own apartment. I worked full time at The Houston Post newspaper and attended law school classes at night. The classical music critic at the newspaper advised me on the purchase of a used piano, which got the most use on Friday evenings as I played out my stress and then put on record albums for free-form dancing.

When I married and had children, I made sure my son and daughter had the opportunities to be involved in activities that interested them. Like his uncles and dad, my son played baseball in elementary school, but my daughter started with gymnastics and switched to dance. I put on tap shoes again to perform in two mother-daughter dances with her at the spring recitals. I will never know if I embarrassed her, but we did get through both recitals without a disaster. At first, my sometimes-shy daughter did not dance like she loved it. I occasionally wondered if she danced just to please me. Then, sometime in her early teen years, the light bulb clicked on, and I proudly watched as her joy suddenly became apparent at a dress rehearsal. She danced with the studio's company team during high school and enrolled in dance classes in college just for fun.

Once the kids were grown, it became time to explore more of what was interesting to me after years of volunteering at the schools. A classmate in the adult tap class at my daughter's studio had told me about a free class for seniors where she danced. It was at the Bay Area Community Center in Clear Lake in southeast Harris County. I finally took a chance and started dancing there in the fall of 2013.

Our instructor, then in her late 70s, had once taught girls in her own studio but was still teaching now with adults – great proof that dancing keeps you young. Her choreography was not so athletic that seniors would hurt themselves, but it was still really cute. The class members weren't at all snobs like my dad once predicted. They were fun, creative people I looked forward to seeing! It took me a year of observing the dances to learn them well enough to perform with the group, usually at nursing homes, where some music and smiles are so welcome. The pandemic shut us down for a while, and the group stayed in touch. When we returned to class, remembering the dances was somewhat harder than climbing back on a bicycle, but most of it has come back.

I finally figured out that tap dancing is a tactile activity, which is probably why I love it so much; it's like running my hands across velvet fabric. Because I got off to a late start, I will never be an expert, and that is okay. At this stage in my life, I am grateful for the opportunity to spend less time on what someone else thinks I should do and more time on what truly brings me pleasure.

* * *

Noula's Story

I grew up in a Greek-speaking family, so when my mother took me to my first dance lesson to learn tap at the age of 5, I spoke only Greek and very little English. During the lesson, as a result of communication barriers, the teacher went up to my mother, watching from the parent's bench, and asked, "Why isn't she moving her feet?" My mother then translated the instructions from the teacher and told me to "copy his feet." It appears I did this well as he seemed to be quite pleased with my response and thought that I was so cute with the potential to learn, he decided to give me private lessons.

Dancing continued through elementary school and a move from Philadelphia, PA, to Wilmington, Delaware. There, my mother found an excellent dance instructor, and my dancing included not only tap but also ballet, toe, some acrobatics (1 yr), and baton twirling. By age 14, through the breadth of experience I picked up along the way, I ended up becoming a teaching assistant for the instructor spending weekends attending classes taught using a live piano player. Recitals were held at the Du-

Pont Hotel Ballroom every year with a full orchestra! The backdrops on stage were professional, and the material for our costumes were ordered from New York.

Although I went through a short phase where I may have lost interest in dance, it wasn't long before I picked up my dance shoes once again and became completely devoted to the art of dance! For the next four summers, I attended dance conventions with my teacher in New York with the prestigious organizations that would host them known as the Dance Masters of America and Dance Educators of America. The days were long and tiring but ever so rewarding. Sometimes as a bonus, these organizations provided me and my instructor free tickets to Broadway shows which helped broaden my horizons that much more!

The ballroom floor was filled with many teachers from all over the country, as the opportunity to train with and learn from the various masters that were brought in for these special sessions in tap and ballet was a great honor and inspiration to all. Some of the guest instructors included names such as Danny Hoctor (tap) and Maria Tallchief (ballet and toe).

At age 17, our family ended up moving back to West Philadelphia, and having developed a true love of dance. I decided to begin my own dance studio in our finished basement. With the help of my parents and brother, we modified the basement to include a large mirror on one wall and a ballet barre on the other. As my father was in the printing business, he would print up advertisements in local papers, and after a few years of my basement classroom teaching, I ended up opening a small dance studio of my own in a nearby community.

At the age of 21, my life changed significantly to include getting married and having four children, but in between, I always found a way to continue dancing and teaching! After a few moves along the East Coast, we ended up settling down permanently in Clear Lake City, a suburb of Houston, Texas. In addition to my own love of dance, I enrolled my 8-year-old daughter in dance lessons at a nearby studio, and I also continued my own dance journey by signing up for adult lessons as well. They quickly learned of my aptitude for dancing and teaching, and soon, I was back to doing what I loved so very much, part-time teaching in many of the dance disciplines I had come to cherish over the years!

After raising my family and spending many summers vacationing in Greece, Line Dancing became a popular form of dance in Texas, which became one more dance discipline to add to my repertoire. In time, I once again began teaching, this time to Seniors. A few friends and acquaintances, knowing of my deep love of and passion for dance, suggested I should share my knowledge with others in the community and, at the age of 65, I ended up teaching Adult Tap and Line Dancing at the Clear Lake Community Center as well as the Friendswood Senior Center. Over the course of the next 20 years, I was extremely blessed to have been able to teach tap and line dancing to so very many seniors who have become lifelong friends in these communities. Not to mention, providing entertainment in the community by having our "Bay Area Chorus Line Tappers" perform at nursing homes and various functions in the area.

With the passing of time, I think back on those early years and am so very grateful for my mother's ingenuity in signing me up for dance lessons at such an early age! As a result, I've been able to reap the rewards of dance throughout my life by meeting so very many beautiful people, all with the very same love of dance.

* * *

Why Couldn't I Just Take Tap!

By Judy

Picture this. December 7, 1941. Me, born on "This Day of Infamy." Pearl Harbor Day. Yes, and my mom was 18 years old. Thank God my mom didn't name me Pearl as the nurses had suggested.

Fast forward. 1946 small town, South Houston, TX, I am 5 years old. Just had my 5th birthday, and what did I get? A baby brother! Also, my first recollection of dance lessons. It was in a very old building and was the City Hall across the street from my grandmother and grand-father's house, where we were living at the time. My dad had just served in the Navy and was returning to a job they held for him when he was drafted.

I remember the classes consisted of Tap, Ballet, and Tumbling. Oh yes, tumbling, never accomplished much. Even standing on my head was a challenge. Ballet, well, pointing my toes gave me such cramps in my feet. But then, TAP. OMG! Yes, I loved it! Even more, on the second story of this old City Hall, that wooden floor echoed. I can still hear it.

Then my mom discovered a new dance studio across the street from our bank, fifteen miles from the house. Back in the day, when you dressed up to go make the weekly deposit inside.

Those classes were also Tap, Ballet, and Tumbling. Must have been a package deal back then. Why couldn't I just take tap? We always had this lady playing the piano for our music. Over and over, we would practice. I didn't mind repeating any practice, just a certain satisfaction. Must have had something to do with my character? I was a very quiet child, and making noise gave me an outlet? Who knows. I remember practicing at home on a little blackboard because my mom didn't want the varnish on the new floors scratched. Very limited.

I remember the shuffle, the flap, and the buffaloe steps were my favorite, and we did a lot of those. Then came the news we were going to perform in a recital. We had to make our own costumes. My grandmother was a seamstress, so I had it made. It was so exciting! It was at the Music Hall in downtown Houston. So much excitement backstage. Then the moment we were up next. My heart was beating a thousand times a minute. I was so scared. Then the curtain opened, and out we went. I was so surprised when my fear instantly disappeared! I couldn't see anything but vast darkness because the spot lights were so bright! I felt like a star. This was going to be my career.

Fast forward. I am 6, almost 7. We moved from my grandmother's into a house my dad and my grandfather built. Money was tight. Mom got a job. No more dance lessons.

Then a great VOID! Years later, married with two children didn't make much time for any dance lessons. Then, at last, retirement 1998! And, no problem filling my time with things other than work. I went to the local senior center to indulge with activities offered.

Hot Dog! Line Dance Classes. Started immediately and loved it! Then Aerobics Classes. During one of these classes, I heard someone mention adult tap dance classes at another senior center. I was on to that immediately! Four members. I made it five. Line dance and aerobics classes soon dropped by the way side as I devoted time to tap exclusively.

I was pleasantly surprised how I remembered those basic shuffle, flap, and buffalo steps. The class began to grow, and the instructor began to teach more advanced routines. We decided to perform as a group in the Senior Olympics. We were on a roll! Gradually, we began to add costumes. A hat, scarf, vest, etc. We were invited to perform at community functions and at nursing homes. Became known as The Silver Star Tap Dance Team and performed for years. I even had the pleasure of a solo on a Royal Caribbean cruise, where I did Give My Regards to Broadway

* * *

My Tap Dance Journey

By Tapdancenana

My journey into tap dancing began when I was six years old. My first-grade teacher was frustrated with my always wanting everything to be perfect behavior and recommended that my parents give me piano or dance lessons to learn that everyone makes mistakes. Dance lessons were less costly, so I was enrolled in Frances Osborne's School of Dance. I received instruction in ballet and tap and fell in love with dance. I favored tap dancing because I loved the sounds my feet made and all the rhythms. I likened myself to Shirley Temple and even got a "TONI" perm to have curls like Shirley's.

As a young teenager, Jimmy Collins, a retired professional ballet dancer with the Boston Ballet Company, started guest teaching at my dance school. At this time, I was taking lessons in ballet and pointe, tap, and jazz. He recognized my acumen in tap and offered me private lessons. It was going to be a stretch on my parents' budget to pay for the lessons, so I took babysitting jobs to help pay for them. Eventually, I transferred to his dance school. I loved the challenging choreography he offered and diligently practiced at home. One evening in class, he took me aside and very matter of factly told me I probably would never dance professionally, I did not have the "body type," but he told me I had what it took to choreograph and teach. Shortly thereafter, a neighbor of my parents opened a dance studio and hired me to teach ballet, tap, jazz, and baton twirling. She paid for my certification training, and I continued to teach for her until I graduated college. Surprise: my undergraduate degree is in Mechanical Engineering with a minor in Mathematics. Math, music, and dance are all related.

Marriage and and raising five children took over my life, so dancing was only for me in the kitchen while cooking or cleaning. By the time my oldest children were off to college, I began training in Taekwondo. My dance background made it easy for me to learn the Poomsae (the choreographed forms for each belt level). Sparring was a different story, however. I recall my son, who was a trainee instructor, tell me not to stand so erect that I was fighting, not dancing! I eventually became an instructor national judge and achieved the rank of 4th degree back belt. In 2006 I won World Champion In weapons form. My form was with double nunchucks. Again my dancing very much influenced my performance.

A move to the Houston, Texas, area brought me back to dance. In 2010 I joined the Bay Area Chorus Line Tappers. Through them, I found an advanced tap class with the Art Park Dance program and the League City Tappers. I currently lead and choreograph for the League City Tappers and continue to attend the advanced tap class in Deer Park.

Tap dancing makes me happy. I enjoy the challenges of learning new steps and creating choreography for the wonderful group of tappers whom have given me the privilege to lead. Tap dancing is ageless and boundless! I intend to keep tapping even into the afterlife! Time to Shuffle off to "Buffalo,"

* * *

My Love Affair with Tap

My love affair with dance began as a small child with the obligatory tap and ballet class once a week. My mother was a dancer, even having her own dance school for a time. She'd already had three sons, so when I came along, it was her great pleasure to get me in dance class at a young age. In addition to the exciting recitals with adorable costumes, I learned rhythm, timing, graceful movements, and even splits and cartwheels! I advanced to dancing on pointe, but my days of dancing school ended when my brother's piano teacher talked me into piano lessons rather than continuing with dance. Her rationale was that I would be able to play the piano the rest of my life, but I wouldn't be able to dance the rest of my life. Too bad she can't see me today still dancing at the age of 71 with no end in sight!

In high school, I was a varsity cheerleader, and cheering in those days was closer to dance than the gymnastic type cheering they do today. I also had social dance with the boys in high school. In college, I majored in Physical Education and Health, so I was required to take square dancing, folk dancing, modern dance and movement, and rhythm classes. Then, of course, throughout my growing up, I watched Dick Clark's American Bandstand and danced with friends as much as possible. After graduation, I took a job at New Brunswick High School in New Jersey, teaching Health and Physical Education.

Fast forward into marriage and two children with dancing mainly at weddings then. Since my husband is Polish, that included many, many polkas. Because of this and other varied exposure to dance in other cultures, I learned to appreciate all dance. Yet I really missed ballet, so rather than putting my preschool daughter in dance class when I was the one who really wanted to be there, I took a job waitressing on weekends to pay for my semi-professional ballet classes once a week at the age of 28. I loved the challenge and quality of these classes, but two years later, my husband got transferred from our home in New Jersey to Houston, Texas. I wanted to resume dance classes but wanted the level of instruction I'd left, not just the local dancing schools. Also, with two young children, I didn't have the luxury of going downtown to classes. A friend told me about a dance program at the University of Houston Clear Lake which is right across the street from my subdivision! I was able to enroll and take five modern dance classes and three ballet classes a week along with the rest of the curriculum. At the end of two years, I received a Master's Degree to boot! In the spring of each of these years, our "final" thesis, if you will, we had to choreograph, set, light, direct, costume, and every other detail of a piece that was all our own. What a fun and enlightening experience that was!

Next, I considered going back to teaching. I was already certified to teach Physical Education, Health, and Dance K - 12 in New Jersey, so I took and passed the required tests to do the same in Texas. I interviewed for a job at an elementary school but then found out that my mom, still in NJ, was diagnosed with Alzheimer's. That consumed the next five years of my life. I had also found an adult tap class nights that I'd started taking for a couple years, but since I had to now travel to NJ so frequently, I stopped.

Years later, I discovered that the community center near me offered a tap class for seniors...for free, no less! Oh, happy day! Shortly after moving to Texas, my husband did come to square dance classes then tried a couple ballroom classes but soon lost interest. To tap, I wouldn't need a partner... perfect! It was amazing to see these women, all older than I, tapping away under the direction of the teacher who was 12 years older than I was! I didn't get much attention from the teacher when I started. It was pretty much "sink or swim." Thankfully I was able to pick up the choreography relatively quickly, but, more importantly, I just loved tapping again! The years went by, I progressed from the back row to the front, actually wore out a pair of tap shoes, and had to buy new ones, and this group continues to this day. Sadly we have lost people but gained others, and hopefully, if this pandemic ever settles down, we will again be able to get back to performing at nursing homes and the like. Inspiringly, the original teacher is still with us and recently had class for us less than three weeks after a heart attack and stroke! I'm very thankful that my passion for dance has been fulfilled in so many creative ways throughout my life! My plan is to dance on!